The Glow Ritual

The information given in this book is for entertainment purposes and should not be treated as a substitute for professional medical advice. Always consult a medical practitioner. Although every effort has been made to ensure that the information in this book was correct at press time, no responsibility is assumed for any loss, damage, or disruption caused by errors or omissions, and no liability is assumed for any damages that may result from the use of this information.

The views expressed in this book are those of the author alone and do not reflect those of That Guy's House Ltd.

This book is a work of creative nonfiction, however, certain elements may have been fictionalized in varying degrees, for various purposes to suit the narrative

The book information is catalogued as follows;
Author Name(s): Jai Koo-Ven
Title: The Glow Ritual
Description; First Edition

Cover Design by Martina Pavlova
Cover Illustration by Martina Pavlova

ISBN: 978-1-914447-49-5 (paperback)
ISBN: 978-1-914447-50-1
 (ebook)

Prepared by That Guy's House Ltd.
www.ThatGuysHouse.com

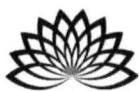

The
GLOW
Ritual

Jai Koo-Ven

Endorsements

"*The GLOW Ritual* is so much more than a self-help book; it's a comprehensive lifestyle guide, providing everything you need to live a 'Glowing Life Of Wellness'! Jai covers everything from chakras to food, meditation to beauty products, and everything in between. This is the sort of book you'll recommend to all of your girlfriends and carry around in your bag with you as a constant companion. So excited to read more from this brilliant new author!"

Jesse Lynn Smart – Senior Editor, Fae Magazine

"Through a chakra journey to wellness, this book will raise your awareness of self, empowering you with the confidence to align with who you would like to become. A treasure trove of wellness and mindset tips."

Claire Stone, Hay House - bestselling author The Female Archangels, Reclaim your Power with the Lost Teachings of the Divine Feminine

The perfect blend of ancient wisdom and ritual with modern day practicality, designed to nourish your mind, body and soul. In my eyes, this is what should be taught in schools so that the young women (and men alike) enter adulthood fully equipped with both the knowledge and the practice that is key to maintaining a healthy, balanced and empowered life amidst the inevitable challenges that arise.

Alie Harwood – Wellness & Confidence Coach at Wellness with Alie

To My Guardian Angel Graham.

As promised, this book is dedicated to you.

I miss you so much and will always love you.

Thank you for always believing in me

and the creation of this book x

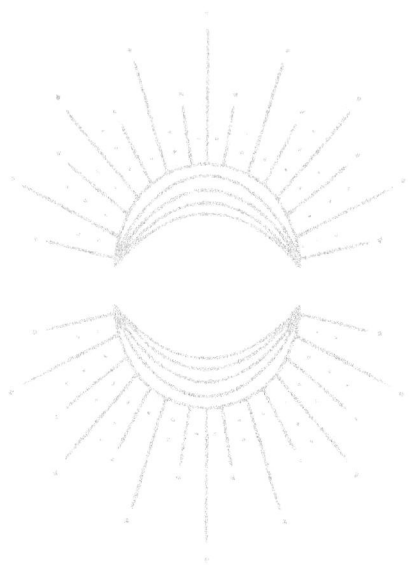

Your Wellness Journey

CHAPTER ONE
ROOT CHAKRA – GLOW WITH GROUNDING

CHAPTER TWO
SACRAL CHAKRA – GLOW WITH THE FLOW

CHAPTER THREE
SOLAR PLEXUS CHAKRA – GLOW WITH JOY

CHAPTER FOUR

PINK HEART CHAKRA – GLOW FROM SELF-LOVE

CHAPTER FIVE

GREEN HEART CHAKRA– GLOW FROM GREENS

CHAPTER SIX

THROAT CHAKRA – GLOW WITH TRUTH

CHAPTER SEVEN

THIRD EYE CHAKRA – GLOW WITH VISION

CHAPTER EIGHT

CROWN CHAKRA – GLOW WITH WISDOM

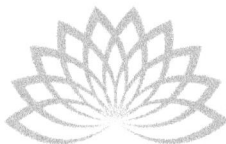

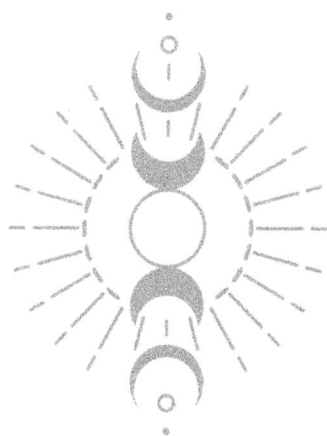

Prologue

MY STORY

Many people live day to day, taking life for granted until something happens to wake you up, like a near death experience or a physical or mental illness, which makes you realise how precious your life really is. In my case, I have experienced all three.

From the age of 12, I had to grow up very quickly due to the fact that I had a brain tumour removed. At that age, you believe that life is limitless and you are invincible, until you are then faced with your own mortality. After most of my brain tumour was removed (I still have some of the tumour remaining), I felt very much like the 'victim' whilst growing up and would often wonder, "Why me?"

I would compare myself to other people's 'perfect life' and often wondered why I had my childhood innocence stripped away. My experience made me feel very fragile, and I felt I could no longer be carefree with my life as I grew older and into adulthood.

This is when I discovered the world of holistic healing and spent the next 15 years dedicating myself to my training and studies. I then started seeing myself as a survivor rather than a victim, and everything changed. Over the years, I made it my mission to support people around the world with my contributions within the wellness industry. Whether it was 1:1 mentoring, my Self-Care Stationery range, my oracle card deck, articles in magazines, my wellness and business programmes and now this book that you hold in your hands; it has all made the difference in healing my clients around the world and now it can help to heal you too.

In order for you to get a greater understanding of my journey and how it can help you, let's start at the beginning …

MY LOVE OF SCENTS

I have always been obsessed with scents from a young age, whether it was the scent of the roses in the garden or the warm and cosy coffee beans brewing in the coffee shop. I would pick flowers in the garden and try to create the next 'Chanel' scent, but obviously on a much cheaper and less impressive scale! As I grew older, I studied aromatherapy and I grew to understand that there was a therapeutic link between scents and wellbeing, and I knew they always made me feel happy.

It was no surprise that years later I would have a career spanning over a decade in luxury fragrance and beauty, training with high-end brands such as *Jo Malone London, L'Occitane* and *Neal's Yard Remedies*.

Even though I loved the work I did, I always felt like there was something missing for me and I really wanted to help people in a different way. So, whilst working for the brands previously mentioned and over the space of 15 years, I studied and gained qualifications in over 27 holistic therapies. I then graduated from an internationally recognized holistic health school as an Accredited Holistic Health & Wellness Coach and I also qualified as a Yin Yoga and Meditation Teacher.

Since that time, I have been featured in national magazines, written *The GLOW Ritual*, launched jewellery, candle and self-care stationery ranges, launched wellness and business programmes to support busy modern women from around the world and created my own oracle card deck. I achieved all of this whilst being a mum to my beautiful nine-year-old little girl.

MY LIFE CHANGED FOREVER

Just after I had my little girl in 2011, I became very ill with post-traumatic stress disorder due to her being premature and nearly dying, and me being in hospital for over six weeks listening to people going into labour and screaming around me.

I tried traditional anti-depressants for a while, but unfortunately nothing worked. So, I turned my attention to healing myself in a holistic way.

That year, I had a spiritual awakening and realized the importance of self-care and holistic wellness for busy women and mothers trying to juggle the demands of everyday life. This led me to create my mentoring and wellness business which specializes in offering self-care solutions and support for the busy modern woman.

My mission is to inspire positivity and promote holistic wellness through my 1:1 mentoring, wellness and business programmes and stationery and crystal ranges in my Self-Care Shop.

On my journey to holistic health and wellness, I found the amount of information out there constantly overwhelming, so I decided to write *The GLOW Ritual* to create a simpler guide to living a *Glowing Life Of Wellness* for busy modern women. Whether you are a student, busy mum, creative entrepreneur, housewife, or maybe all of these, this book is for you, and it will take you on a wonderful 31-day wellness journey.

So, allow me to introduce you to *The GLOW Ritual* and explain how it will change your life …

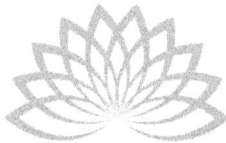

What is a Ritual?

I have always loved the word 'ritual' - there is something so mysterious and mystical about the word that makes it feel sacred.

For years whilst researching this book, I studied various rituals from around the world, from Buddhist rituals to habit rituals, from eating rituals to beauty rituals. One thing they all had in common was that a 'ritual' contributed to you becoming a better version of yourself.

This is the definition of a ritual from Wikipedia:

> *A ritual is a sequence of activities involving gestures, words, actions, or objects, performed in a sequestered place and according to a set sequence. Rituals may be prescribed by the traditions of a community including a religious community. Rituals are characterized, but not defined, by formalism, traditionalism, invariance, rule-governance, sacral symbolism and performance.*

Rituals can help us remember a family member who has died, celebrate a new life coming into the world, or celebrate important holidays. Symbolic actions that are repeated and are part of your routine – whether this is daily, weekly, or yearly – are known as a ritual.

Here are some examples of rituals from around the world:

An example of a birth ritual is when a Christian family celebrate the birth of a new child and have their baby baptised to wash away original sins.

All around the world, different cultures ritualise marriage through various ways. Some marriages may be religious and take place in a church or a temple, whereas other couples may elope to get married and have a private service.

Another ritual that people celebrate is New Year. A New Year symbolises new beginnings and new hope for a better year. We get a renewed sense of energy when we start a new year, like we are starting a new chapter in our lives as we close the book on our past year.

DISCOVERING YIN YOGA

I love bringing rituals into my life, as they help me feel grounded. When I feel overwhelmed or lost, my daily rituals help me to stay on track with my wellness goals. In the past, my rituals have been my saviour when my anxiety has hit, or when I have felt confused or lost about my future. Rituals are my go-to; they help me quieten my mind, reset myself and put my best self out into the world. One of my favourite rituals to do when I am feeling anxious or uptight is to practice Yin Yoga. I love Yin Yoga - it is a slow style of yoga which incorporates traditional Chinese medicinal principles with body postures (asanas) that are each held for a few minutes. Yin Yoga helps to stretch and target the deep connective tissue between the muscles with the aim to improve flexibility, exercising the joint and bone areas. It also helps to increase the circulation in the joints.

You will see Yin Yoga featured in my wellness membership, as well as in this book. There are also many different YouTubers you can follow to find out more and who can also support you on your journey, including *Boho Beautiful, Yoga with Kassandra*, and *Yoga with Adriene*.

DISCOVERING MEDITATION

Another way that I practice my daily rituals is through meditation; I light a candle and sit in a quiet space in my home and listen to a meditation on my membership or I enjoy the silence. This allows me to have 10-15 minutes of quiet time for myself where I can train my awareness and attention to feel mentally clear and emotionally calm. You can also find an abundance of different meditations on YouTube or through applications like *Headspace* or *Calm* and I will explain about the power of meditation further on in this book.

From this brief introduction, you can see the benefits of having rituals in your life and how they can keep you spiritually grounded. With this as a foundation of understanding, we can now move onto the next section, **What Are Chakras?**

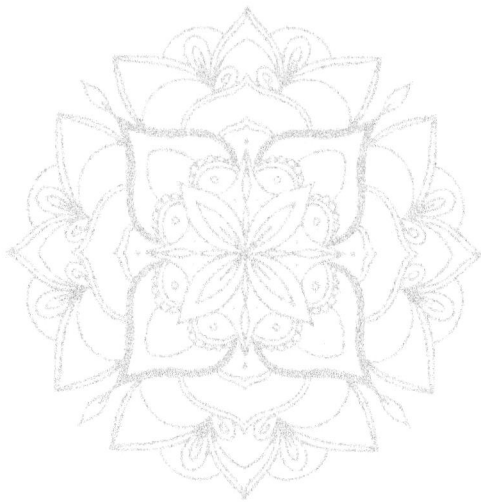

What are Chakras?

Learning to understand Chakras can often be quite difficult if you are a complete beginner. So, I have tried to explain it as easy as I can for you in this book to help you understand yourself better from an energetic level and know when you are off balance.

Chakras are the concentrated energy centres within the body. The Sanskrit term *Chakra* means 'wheel' or 'disk' - it is derived from the root word *cakra*. The Chakras act as spinning wheels of energy or light. Each Chakra has the loving responsibility of emanating energy around our body to keep us functioning at optimal levels. When a Chakra is not functioning properly, it can become blocked, and illness is more prone to occur. How we feel emotionally is greatly dependent on the Chakras within our body and what is out of balance. When we are feeling depressed, we may not be taking in the maximum amount of energy that we need. We may not nourish our body with the proper foods and nutrients, and so, we are depleting our energy levels. Feelings such as anger and jealously can also cause blocks to a healthy energetic flow. These psycho-power centres and energy channels are known as 'the subtle body'. Here is the definition of the subtle body from the Chopra website:

> *The subtle body is in a different realm than the physical body and the mind, but has a powerful impact on the body, mind, and entire system. The human body system thrives*

when the Chakras and the nadis are open and prana, or life force, is allowed to move throughout the system with ease. Any kind of disturbance or disease in the body, mind, or spirit can cause blockage and imbalance. The goal is harmony. So, if you've been feeling out of sorts, take a closer look at your Chakras to investigate what's going on and begin to find balance.

By understanding the Chakras and your energy, you can work on your physical, emotional, mental and spiritual health. There are actually 114 Chakras in the body, but we are most familiar with the seven main ones.

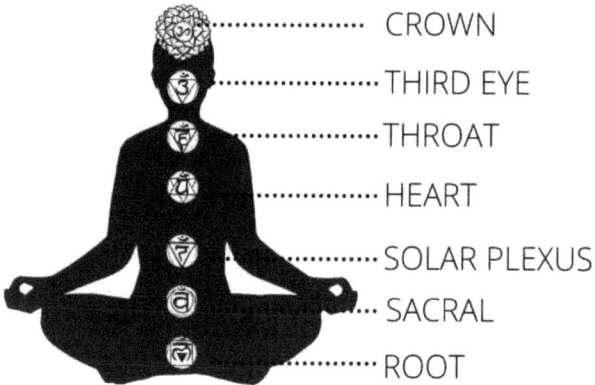

CROWN
THIRD EYE
THROAT
HEART
SOLAR PLEXUS
SACRAL
ROOT

THERE ARE 7 MAIN CHAKRAS

ROOT CHAKRA (MULADHARA)
Strength & Grounding

SACRAL CHAKRA (SVADHISTHANA)
Freedom & Creativity

SOLAR PLEXUS CHAKRA (MANIPURA)
Joy & Abundance

HEART CHAKRA (ANAHATA)
(Pink/ Feminine)
Self- Love, Beauty & Surrender
(Green/ Masculine)
Balance & Protection

THROAT CHAKRA (VISHUDDHA)
Truth & Integrity

THIRD EYE CHAKRA (AJNA)
Clarity & Wisdom

CROWN CHAKRA (SAHASRARA)
Calm & Wisdom

HOW DO YOU KNOW WHEN YOUR CHAKRAS ARE OUT OF BALANCE?

You will know if your Chakras are out of balance because you may have negative recurring patterns in your life, suffer from certain issues, or maybe even have health ailments. For example, you might keep getting a sore throat or have problems expressing yourself verbally. If this is the case, then your throat Chakra may be out of balance. You may have Chakras that are misaligned, with one being underactive and another being overactive, which can make life feel challenging. This is a great example of where yoga has a huge influence on how we feel and can help us balance our Chakras. Because the Chakra system is internal and unseen, it takes a lot of personal awareness to know when your Chakras are out of balance. We can't see when we are out of alignment, but we can feel it deep inside parts of our body. Chakras are part of the energetic body, or subtle body; therefore, it is the energy that lies within us that connects, moves and creates who we are.

YOGA FOR BALANCE

Yoga can help you balance your Chakras and go with the flow of life. It helps you stay grounded and relaxed when the world may feel stormy around you. It creates a peaceful mind in a world which may feel chaotic at times. Therefore, many people practice yoga all around the world because it not only revitalizes your body, but it works on your mind and spirit too.

QUICK REFERENCE GUIDE FOR CHAKRAS

Life is beautiful when your Chakras are in balance. You can experience an immense feeling of joy and fullness in all aspects of your life including mental, physical, emotional, *and* a full mind, body and soul connection. Everything in our life just flows. Life feels graceful, easy and fluid.

As you read through the chapters and 31 daily rituals in this book, you'll see I have delved into each Chakra individually to make it easier for you to understand and to make your daily ritual practice easier, too. As there is a lot of content in this book, some of the daily rituals do also cross over into different Chakras, but I have tried to keep them specific to each Chakra where possible.

So, now you have a greater understanding of my background story and what both rituals and Chakras are, let me introduce you to…

THE GLOW RITUAL

**A Modern Woman's Guide to a
Glowing Life Of Wellness**

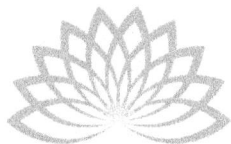

What is The Glow Ritual?

WRITING MY WAY TO WELLNESS

I always wanted to write a book that would empower my readers to live healthy, happy and holistic lives. When I started writing this book, my friends would ask me, 'What is **The GLOW Ritual**?' So, here is my answer …

The GLOW Ritual is a 31-day self-care guide that contains all the tips, tools and holistic advice that I have used over many years to heal myself both mentally and physically. **The GLOW Ritual** is both the method and the goal of living a **Glowing Life Of Wellness** through:

Gratitude & **G**et Creative
Live Holistically
Organise Your Life
Wellness Rituals

Over 15 years, I have read hundreds of self-help books, and studied and qualified as an International Holistic Expert (with over 27 qualifications and counting!)

I often used to wish that I could collate all the information that I have learnt over the years and create my own my own spiritual guide to give me positive guidance and motivation through the hard times, or give me a '**GLOW** up' when I needed it.

RECOVERING FROM POST TRAUMATIC STRESS DISORDER

I had the idea for **The GLOW Ritual** back in 2011 when I was diagnosed with Post-Traumatic Stress Disorder (PTSD) after the birth of my daughter (which I started to explain in the Prologue).

I had been in hospital for about six weeks as my waters broke early and there was a high risk of infection. At night, all I could hear were women going into labour and screaming in the beds next to me. After I came out of hospital, I would try to sleep at night and all I could hear was the same screaming, or if I was in a public place and heard shouting or screaming, I would have a major panic attack. I knew that I no longer felt like me but put that down to being a new (exhausted) mum who was very sleep deprived. However, upon visiting the doctors, they diagnosed me with PTSD and were quick to prescribe with me anti-depressants. Now, I was never one to take pills and I am not against anyone else taking them if they work for you, but for me, I have always opted to heal myself the natural way. Yet, in this instance, I was so desperate to get better that I would have tried anything. I started taking those pills daily and felt like an absolute zombie; I felt sick and dizzy, and they made me very physically ill and low on energy.

So, I then went back to the doctors and they prescribed me another type of anti-depressants. They were better in the sense that I felt a little more normal, but after five or six weeks of taking these pills, I slowly realized that this medication was now the remote control of my life. I had no control because I was reliant on them to make me 'happy'. Sadly, they did not make me happy but rather numb to my own life. It felt like the pills did not deal with the mental trauma that I was going through, instead it was just putting a plaster on it to cushion the blow of anxiety and sadness I was feeling every day.

Other than happiness with my family, I felt nothing; no joy, no sadness, nothing. My life outside of my family just felt empty. Luckily, I was overjoyed at being a mum and this is what helped me get through my bad days.

CHOOSING ANOTHER WAY

I often would think that there must be another way. The pills would just mask my emotions, but not actually cure my suffering. If I felt more anxious, I could not just pop another pill. If I felt sad, the pill would not make me happier. It was then I realized that this was not the right answer for me. The pills made me feel reliant on them. I had horrible side effects when I started taking them but then if I stopped I had the fear of the withdrawal symptoms, so it was a vicious cycle. So, you end up feeling trapped either way and all you want to do is get better.

However, despite my fear, I decided no matter what, I would get off those pills and find other ways to heal myself. I was on a low dose anyway, so I slowly reduced my dosage and then cut them out completely. This is just my story and what worked for me. **However, I do not advise this for anyone that is reading this book and strongly advise you to see a medical professional for advice on your own mental health.**

After about a week of coming off the pills, I no longer felt in that 'fog' that they can put you in and I felt in control of my life again. It was then that I started studying and reading more and more about holistic living and how to heal yourself in natural ways. I was fascinated by this wonderful world of spirituality and wellness and how I could lead a happier life and have it in abundance.

To begin my journey back to health and wellness, I started out by setting myself little 'Wellness Tasks' every day. At first, I put pressure on myself, and I would write things down like 'Do a one-hour workout', when emotionally and energetically I could only last 10-15 minutes. So, I took the pressure off myself and instead of calling them 'Tasks' I would call it 'My Happy Hour'. I started off writing 3-6 things down that would make me holistically happy and healthy and I would make sure that I would spend between 5-10 minutes each day doing as many things as possible in My Happy Hour. I used this as the foundation of my days and bit by bit, day by day, I finally grew stronger both mentally and physically. I fuelled this 'Happy Hour' with positivity, and it allowed me to have a great start to my day. It made me feel like I had really achieved something and it allowed me to stay grounded and connected to my wellbeing. Through the success of this routine, I renamed it *The GLOW Ritual* (*Glowing Life of Wellness*). To me it was the perfect name, as I love candles and the soft glow of candlelight. *The GLOW Ritual* is that inner and outer glow that you get when you are looking after your wellbeing.

MUM'S BABY STEPS

In my darkest moments when I had PTSD, I started to write poems to help me through the dark times. I kept them all in a book that I called Mum's Baby Steps and it was my journey of getting my life back to wellness after having PTSD. As I started to get better, I realized that I did not want to write a book for my readers which was filled with doom and gloom. Instead, I wanted to write a book of truth, hope, empowerment and inspiration to help you to live the best life you could ever live and support you in your journey back to wellness. I also felt that it would be of some comfort for my readers to know that in the darkest moments there is always light at the end of that dark tunnel.

The GLOW Ritual teaches you a *Glowing Life of Wellness* through little rituals you can do each day to help lift your mood, understand holistic living, and write your way to wellness.

No matter what scenario you are faced with, *The GLOW Ritual* will provide you with everything you need to move forward - 31 daily self-care rituals to help you keep on track throughout the month and Chakra guidance to help you to stay balanced. It is your own spiritual toolbox of tips and tricks to help you feel in control of your life. Keep it with you for inspiration when you feel stuck and need motivation, and remember that no matter what, you will get better if you change your mindset. If you want more support on your self-care journey, then you can also apply to my wellness programme which includes access to *The Mind Spa Membership*, where there is a *31-Day Self-Care Challenge*, as well as lots of daily rituals that you can create on your own with help from me and my team of Holistic Experts.

It is my mission to help as many people as possible understand that your wellness starts and ends with you. You must find what works for you and not rely on other people or materialistic things to make you happy. This is when I found my true happiness.

The GLOW Ritual is that feeling you get inside of you when you do something positive in your life or are in a creative flow state. Think of the glow from a candle when it burns. When that candle burns, it's like your problems are melting away.

At the end of each chapter and each day, there are rituals for you to complete so that you can apply the lessons in the chapters to your life and write your way to wellness through journaling.

At the end of each chapter in this book, there are also crystal and essential oil recommendations because there are so many times when you may feel you need a crystal or an aromatherapy oil for support, but do not really know what they do. These recommendations make it easy for you to understand what you need and how it can help you.

EMBRACING *THE GLOW RITUAL*

The GLOW Ritual is to help you keep a positive focus, no matter what life throws your way. To look after your wellbeing each day, just remember to add *The GLOW Ritual* into your life.

Gratitude & Get Creative
Live Holistically
Organise Your Life
Wellness Rituals

Doing one of each of these rituals each day will help to bring you back into balance.

Once you know your path, you can easily be guided back towards it. When you do not have a clear focus in your life or your days, this is when depression and anxiety can easily take over and you can lose your feeling of purpose. I strongly believe that my purpose, besides being a mother and a wife, is to help thousands of people all over the world to discover ***The GLOW Ritual*** and live their best, holistically beautiful, boho lives.

The 31-days of Wellness Rituals in this book are to support you with your own daily ***GLOW Ritual*** so you can learn different elements of holistic living, writing rituals, wellness rituals, and organised living that you can add into your life each day. These 31-Days of Rituals are broken down into eight main chapters:

CHAPTER 1 – Root Chakra – ***GLOW*** WITH GROUNDING
CHAPTER 2 – Sacral Chakra – ***GLOW*** WITH THE FLOW
CHAPTER 3 – Solar Chakra – ***GLOW*** WITH JOY
CHAPTER 4 – Pink Heart Chakra – ***GLOW*** WITH SELF-LOVE
CHAPTER 5 – Green Heart Chakra – ***GLOW*** WITH GREENS
CHAPTER 6 – Throat Chakra – ***GLOW*** WITH TRUTH
CHAPTER 7 – Third Eye – ***GLOW*** WITH VISION
CHAPTER 8 – Crown Chakra – ***GLOW*** WITH WISDOM

So, now let's begin ***The GLOW Ritual*** and your 31-day journey to your ***Glowing Life Of Wellness*** …

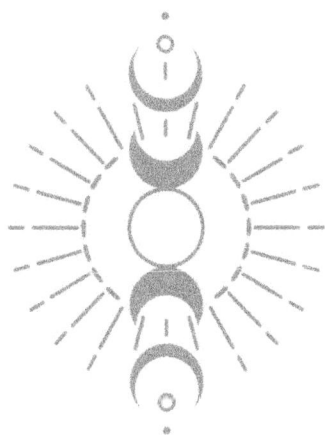

Glow with Grounding

❁

CHAPTER

One

ROOT CHAKRA

THE ROOT CHAKRA

The Root Chakra is also referred to as *Muladhara* and is the Chakra for strength and grounding. *Mula* means 'root' and *Adhara* means 'base' or 'support'. The Root Chakra has a gorgeous lotus flower with four petals as its symbol.

The Root Chakra can help you to feel safe and secure in your physical and emotional needs. It triggers the survival instincts within you and that feeling of your fight or flight response to things happening around you.

As the Root Chakra is the first of the chakras, it helps you to create a more stable foundation for the chakras above it A solid foundation builds stability in your life and therefore it is vital to keep a healthy Root Chakra, so you can live a stable, secure and grounded life.

WHERE IS THE ROOT CHAKRA LOCATED?

The Root Chakra is located at the base of your spine.

WHAT COLOUR IS THE ROOT CHAKRA?

Red.

HOW WILL I FEEL IF THIS CHAKRA IS BALANCED?

- You will feel vitality for life
- You will feel grounded
- You are rooted in your own energy and are not

influenced by other people's thoughts, feelings, actions or words

- You remain centred and balanced in stressful situations, which normally cause people to feel anxious and overwhelmed

- You can easily maintain healthy relationships and authentic connections

- You are in touch with your body and are aware of the sensations of discomfort or pain

- You are connected to Mother Nature, which helps to cool your anger and absorb your anxiety

- You feel at home and safe in this world

- You have a true sense of belonging and appreciate the gift of being alive

- You have faith and trust in the unknown and feel less fear

- You can manifest stability and security because you are more organised and efficient

- You never lose things or feel chaotic

- You surrender your worries because you trust that everything will work out for the best

- Being in stillness is not a worry to you, as it allows you to be able to hear the guidance from your intuition

HOW MIGHT I FEEL IF I AM OUT OF BALANCE?

- You may experience depression and anxiety and have

nightmares

- You can develop problems with your lower limbs and hip pain

- An overactive Root Chakra may make you feel like you have a lack of energy, feel greed and materialism, be overweight, have anger issues or a sense of being headstrong

- When you are deficient in the Root Chakra energy, you may also feel insecure, restless, disconnected, underweight or have lack of discipline

SELF-LOVE WAYS TO GET BACK IN BALANCE

- Wearing or visualizing red when in meditation

- When you are unbalanced, it is important to understand the root of your problem so, you can work through it fully

- Take part in yoga class to balance your Root Chakra through my membership programme or by watching a YouTube video

- Take a walk-in nature, barefoot if you can

- Pamper your feet through a relaxing foot massage or pedicure

DAY 1
A RITUAL FOR STRENGTH

'Champions aren't made in gyms. Champions are made from something they have deep inside them – a desire, a dream, a vision.'
Muhammad Ali

LOOKING AFTER YOUR MENTAL HEALTH

My journey into Holistic Health and Wellness started 15 years ago, however, I truly discovered it and the healing power it had on my life 10 years ago.

Just after my daughter was born and I was recovering from PTSD, whenever I felt sad and my emotions were up and down, I would write poems about my feelings. I only wrote the poems for me and, as I mentioned earlier, I called my book *Mum's Baby Steps*.

Like a child taking their first steps into their new world, your journey back to good mental health can feel the same way, no matter what you are going through. You feel fragile, scared and unsteady on your feet. Just one wrong footing can knock you sideways and make you feel like giving up. Yet, every day, you still stand up tall, ready to try again, and step by step you gain the confidence to keep moving forward.

Life is unsteady at times, and it is unpredictable, so when you know that you have tools at hand to support you whenever you need them, you never feel alone on your journey back to wellbeing.

During my darkest times, I could not see so far into the future. I knew that I just had to take it day by day, enjoy my new baby and learn how to heal myself again. So, I would plan achievable tasks for the next 24 hours and that would be my focus each day. As I achieved more, I grew mentally stronger, and it gave me the confidence to add more things to my list without being overwhelmed. Beyond my beautiful baby and my husband, it also gave me my own purpose.

PTSD can make you feel depressed. I often felt incredibly conflicted; I was so happy being a mummy and a wife and it was the best gift in the world, but the PTSD was making every other aspect of my life sad. I gave everything I could to my daughter and husband, but I had nothing left to give to myself. I had lost my passion and purpose for all other things apart from them. At night when they slept soundly, I would cry myself to sleep and I would feel very alone

Yet, when I started writing my *Mum's Baby Steps* poems, I started to realise that just like my little girl, I needed to take baby steps too. So, I started off small - *Today, I will read a page of a book, Tomorrow I will make a fruit salad*, etc.

When you experience any trauma in life, it is hard for your brain to forget what happened. However, PTSD trauma replays over and over in your head like a broken tape recorder, and anything can trigger it. This then can materialise into crying, depressive thoughts and anxiety.

When I felt off track, the little goals I set myself really did help me to feel more like me again, and slowly I added more and more things to my happy list to keep myself motivated. I learnt that no matter how small the step was that I was taking to get back to health, any step was better than none. Inaction would cause procrastination and loss of direction, and this would make me feel more depressed. Social media did not help either.

THE COMPARISON GAME

Unfortunately, with social media nowadays portraying 'perfect lives', with fake filtered pictures and rented homes for a day that people pretend are their own, our version of a 'dream life' can feel unachievable. You can scroll and see a pregnant lady that has just given birth, back to a Size 6 within a week. The 'perfect woman', in the 'perfect life', with the 'perfect husband' and the 'perfect house', etc. You will feel quite content with your life and then scroll on your social feed and feel rubbish about yourself within an instant. Seeing someone on a luxury holiday, when your days are filled with dirty nappies or working in an office, can make you no longer feel good about where you are in your life.

Unfortunately, a lot of the time, it is all fake, fake, fake. You never know what goes on behind the scenes as all you see is a single two second snapshot of someone's life that they have chosen to share with the world, which is often filtered and edited. This is one of the very reasons why there is a massive issue with social media and mental health. We end up playing the comparison game with something that is not real or achievable. Therefore, many times I have wanted to get off social media myself and, maybe one day, I will. I feel conflicted because the work I do dictates that I need to be 'visible' to the world. However, to me, too much visibility is vanity, and I am not here on this world to get followers, likes and comments. I am here to help and support people that want to improve their wellbeing. The problem is that healing takes time, and many people want a 'quick fix' solution.

THE QUICK FIX SOLUTION

One thing that I find infuriating at times is the modern

age 'Quick Fix Solution'. Most people want things in an instant. *Lose weight in two weeks, earn a million in a month, get rich quick*!

The graft and determination is gone for most people, as they just want to be 'Instafamous'. The truth is, there is no 'Quick Fix Solution' that is sustainable. Yes, you might get rich quick but lack a positive money mindset and then you lose it all. You might go to the doctor because you are depressed, then take the pill and feel a little better. Yet, a week or a month later you are still left with the problem that you never dealt with because you did not learn to manage it properly.

If you are determined to get what you want, then you will do anything to achieve that, no matter how long it takes. Looking after your mental health is a lifetime commitment, not a 'Quick Fix Solution'. Running a successful business is the same and so is losing weight. Yes, the weight might fall off quickly, but if you don't sustain that weight loss, then you will easily put that weight back on again. Similarly, if you do not sustain your business, then it will fail.

The best advice I have for you today is little and often, every day. You are better off doing 20 sit-ups everyday than doing 100 in a day then not bothering for a month. By creating these little healthy habits, it is easier for you to sustain your goals and health and achieve vitality in all areas of your life.

As I mentioned before, these little positive seeds that you plant will not seem like much when you first get started, but they will soon blossom into something beautiful. For example, you will see your body changing, you will finish that book you always wanted to write, or you will launch a business you always wanted to create.

Having a healthy workout routine is great for your physical health but it will help you grow mentally strong too.

Keep one foot in front of the other and keep moving forwards each day. It all starts with just one little step.

So, this now leads us to today's ***The GLOW Ritual*** **for Strength...**

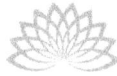

THE GLOW RITUAL
FOR STRENGTH

GRATITUDE & GET CREATIVE
Journaling Prompts

Write down in your journal:

- No matter whether you are feeling happy or sad, answer the question, "What is the next thing I can do to feel better?"
- Set yourself little goals that you believe you can achieve today
- Write down 5 things you are grateful for today

LIVE HOLISTICALLY
Life Lessons

- With simple habits, little and often, you can achieve your goals
- Don't compare yourself to anyone but you
- Keep working on keeping your Root Chakra balanced in order to create a solid and strong foundation
- Looking after your mental health will lead to happiness

ORGANISE YOUR LIFE
Get Organised

The Root Chakra is about building stable foundations for our growth, health and happiness through grounding. Today, spend 20-minutes in your garden, balcony or terrace and organise a wonderful space where you can relax in. If you do not have a garden, then take a 20-minute walk in nature to organise your thoughts and feelings.

WELLNESS RITUALS
Time For Self-Care

Try a new type of workout to boost your mental and physical strength, something different like yoga or pilates, then follow this with a lovely chilled out meditation to balance your Root Chakra.

I would love to see *The GLOW Ritual* that you have decided to create for yourself today.

Don't forget to also tick each part of *The GLOW Ritual* **off each day to support you in living your** *Glowing Life Of Wellness*:

Gratitude & **G**et Creative
Live Holistically
Organise Your Life
Wellness Rituals

Share with me www.jaikooven.co.uk

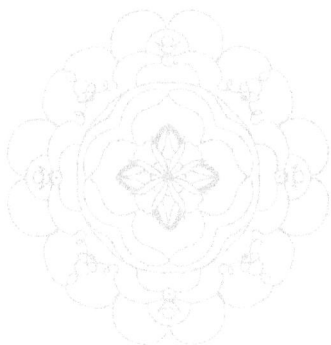

DAY 2
A RITUAL FOR GROUNDING

'Very little grows on jagged rock. Be grounded. Be crumbled so wildflowers will come up where you are.'
Rumi

BUILDING FROM THE GROUND UP

You often hear of people saying things like, "My life is falling apart", "I'm building from the ground up" or "I have hit rock bottom" and they are often associated with negative or traumatic circumstances or often trying to start a business. However, when we change our mindset about this situation, we can find that what is falling apart is actually falling into place for our highest good and we can then embrace a whole new beginning.

THE TREE OF LIFE

The Tree of Life is a spiritual symbol that signifies our personal growth, development, strength, beauty, wisdom and uniqueness. In many different cultures it is also recognized as the symbol for eternal life and immortality. As the tree establishes its roots and grounds itself into the Earth, it creates a strong foundation where its branches can grow strong, striving to grow bigger and better as it reaches for the sky.

Our Root Chakra acts in the same way for our spiritual growth. If we have weak roots, we are unable to connect fully to good foundations and flourish as we should.

As I have been writing this book, it has taken me on

such a journey; from a little seed of an idea, something beautiful has slowly blossomed into life.

Therefore, **The GLOW Ritual** begins here right at the Root Chakra. You can build a whole new foundation for yourself, one that will support you in creating the life you want by establishing a solid foundation.

TIME IN NATURE

Getting out in nature and breathing in the fresh air is so important for our wellbeing. Nature not only allows us to 'get rooted with our Root Chakra', but it allows us to experience the following things:

- Reconnect to Mother Nature
- Control depression
- Reduce anxiety
- Help us to get exercise
- Help improve immunity and memory
- Make us feel happy
- Improve our athletic performance

There is also a term called 'Nature Therapy', aka 'Ecotherapy', that describes a broad group of techniques or treatments to help an individual's mental and physical wellbeing by being within nature.

Another term used often is 'nature bathing'. Nature bathing comes from the Japanese concept *Shinrin-Yoku*, which means 'forest bathing' or 'relaxing in a forest atmosphere'. You don't need to get naked or wear a swimsuit to nature bathe. The idea is that you are 'bathing' in the energy and clear, clean air of the woods.

So, next time you are feeling anxious or depressed, instead of a hot bath, take some mindful minutes away from your house and bathe in nature.

HOW DOES NATURE HELP YOU FEEL GROUNDED?

Being in nature helps you connect to the earth and is a great therapeutic technique that can help you feel a lot happier with a strong sense of wellbeing. It can also help to alleviate stress and boosts your immune system. Having contact with the soil on your bare feet or hands, transfers healing microbes through your body. This is because nature is peaceful and calming and does not judge us.

Our modern society is all about rushing, materialism, stress and always wanting and doing more with an endless and ever-growing to-do list. Nature gives us the time-out we need to reset our minds and reconnect with our roots. When stress and the lack of feeling grounded takes over, and we start to spend too much time indoors and on technology, we can lose our connection to ourselves and the earth and what truly matters for our health and wholeness.

As nature is endless and nurturing, to become grounded, you must immerse yourself in nature daily. Learn from it and draw inspiration from this amazing, calming and serene energy.

When you take time to slow down, it is amazing what you can learn about your life and your surroundings. Taking time out of your day to practice yoga in nature is something really special that you can add to your day. It can be truly transformational as you get to experience the deep connection with nature and the sense of calm in your mind. Yoga is all about working on training our bodies and mind to move with ease and be calm. Moving and breathing whilst in nature, you can feel fully connected as you observe the colours and the calm of your peaceful environment.

If yoga is not for you, there are other alternatives I have found that are equally therapeutic. One being to take a journal with you outdoors, sit in nature and write about your feelings. Or you can take a book and immerse yourself in a beautiful story in your tranquil surroundings.

Nature is a wonderful nurturer for keeping you grounded, and the best thing is that it is free. Take a step out into nature each day and just breathe.

So, this now leads us to today's *The GLOW Ritual* **for Grounding…**

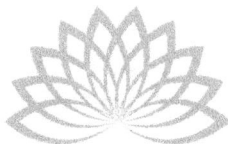

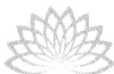

THE GLOW RITUAL
FOR GROUNDING

GRATITUDE & GET CREATIVE
Journaling Prompts

Write in your journal today:

- What will help you feel more grounded in life?
- How can you add time in nature into your daily rituals?
- What are 5 things you are grateful for today?

LIVE HOLISTICALLY
Life Lessons

- Spending time in nature helps you to stay more grounded and connected to the earth.
- The Tree of Life is a great symbol of spiritual growth and personal development.
- By changing your mindset, you are able to create good and solid foundations for your health, happiness and growth.

ORGANISE YOUR LIFE
Get Organised

Today, spend 20-minutes creating a foundation for your daily routines. Are you currently feeling disorganised, or would you like to create more healthy habits? Starting today, work on establishing your new routine to act as a strong foundation for your days.

WELLNESS RITUALS
Time For Self-Care

Go for a 20-minute walk in nature without your phone or other technology. Take a book, a journal or your yoga mat. Walk barefoot on the earth and connect to the nature surrounding you. You can go in your garden, on a beach, or have a walk in the woods. Whatever it is you decide to do, just fully connect to nature and be mindful of everything around you. What can you see? What can you hear? What do you feel? Find a special tree, sit under it and meditate or do yoga. Feel the flow of nature's energy around you.

I would love to see *The GLOW Ritual* you have decided to create for yourself today.

Don't forget to also tick each part of *The GLOW Ritual* off each day to support you in living your *Glowing Life Of Wellness*:

Gratitude & **G**et Creative
Live Holistically
Organise Your Life
Wellness Rituals

Share with me www.jaikooven.co.uk

DAY 3
A RITUAL FOR LETTING GO

'In the process of letting go, you will lose many things from the past, but you will find yourself.'
Deepak Chopra

Today's ritual can be done over a week or a day. There is a lot of information, but it will make you feel amazing when you have a decluttered mind and home.

DECLUTTERING DETOX

Being a Cancerian, my home (or shell, so to speak!) is extremely important to me. How it looks and feels affects me on a very strong emotional and spiritual level. If my house starts to get very messy, I can feel my anxiety levels go up and I can start to feel very frustrated with my surroundings. When I walk into a room, I want to feel at peace and calm. I want to be able to walk over to my sofa and feel like I can relax, not having to step over a million things to get there!

I remember once watching a programme called *Hoarding: Buried Alive*, all about people who live in extremely messy and cluttered houses 24/7. The homeowners are often suffering from some anxiety or depression because of it, and it is affecting their social life too. They have no energy to clear the mess and are so embarrassed by it they do not want anyone friends or family to come over. Often, they have not had anyone visit for up to 10 years.

It is an endless circle until the helpers on the show work their magic and reset the home to a wonderful tranquil space again. The owner often finds the process of decluttering very stressful. This is because everything we own holds our energy. So, when you have an extremely messy space that you don't want to go into, it is because it's holding negative energy until it is cleared. It kind of acts like a blocked Chakra. When your house is finally tidy again your energy will reset and the positive energy can move around your home again.

CHILDHOOD TRAUMA

Another reason why I realise that my home is so important to me, is because of my childhood memories. When I was in the first couple of years at senior school, me and my mum lived in a two-bedroom council flat in Coventry. One day, I had gotten dressed to go to school and opened the door and there was a man passed out in the main communal hall. My mum and I quickly shut the door, and I could not go to school that day. At the time, unbeknown to me and my mum, we lived next door to a drug dealer, so the reason why the man was on the floor was because of the drugs he had taken.

After this happened, it really affected how I felt about my home and me inviting my friends back into what should have been 'my safe place'. I felt embarrassed and I just wanted to leave. I would make excuses as to why they could not come over. However, due to my mum being a single parent, we had no money to move so we had no choice but to stay there for a little while longer.

I realized that, as I got older, I held onto those feelings of wanting my home to feel like a safe place. I need to feel like I can breathe in my space and not be surrounded by clutter. This is part of understanding and healing my inner child, which I talk more about in Chapter 6.

That is why one of the steps of **The GLOW Ritual** is '*Organise Your Life*'. Having a daily ritual to keep your home and life in order works wonders for your wellbeing. It does not have to be neat all the time, but a tidy house keeps a tidy mind. So, if you can keep your housekeeping in check, then your mind will thank you.

TIDY HOUSE, TIDY MIND

I recommend reading Marie Kondo's *The Life-Changing Magic of Tidying Up*. It's a great book for anyone that is not into tidying or decluttering. She teaches her readers her 'KonMari Method' which is to keep only 'what sparks joy' - with this mindset you can declutter and keep a tidy home easier.

She also helps you run through the process of how to declutter. We have always been taught that you should declutter per room, but Marie shows you that it is better to declutter by category e.g., books, papers, clothes, etc.

I am now trained and certified in the 'KonMari Method' and, along with my expertise in holistic living and wellbeing, I feel it has been a huge benefit in my life and my clients too.

When you declutter anything in your life, whether it is your computer, your home or your mind, you are getting rid of what no longer serves you and opening yourself up to new opportunities to live in a lovely home, in lovely surroundings, with a clear and calm mind.

OTHER WAYS TO ORGANISE YOUR HOME

Another way that you can transform your space is by researching Feng Shui. According to Wikipedia:

'Feng Shui, is a pseudoscientific traditional practice from China, which claims to use energy forces to harmonise individuals with their surrounding environment. The term Feng Shui literally translates as 'wind-water' in English.'

Another way to make your home a happy space is to 'Hygge Your Home'. *Hygge* (pronounced hoo-ga) is from the Danish culture and is all about creating cosy comfort in your home. From candles, rugs and meals with family, to the much-needed digital detox, it combines the mood of cosiness and comfort with feelings of wellness and contentment. It is all about having good things in your life with good people. This explains why the Danes are some of the happiest people in the world.

DECLUTTER YOUR HOME

No matter whether you choose to incorporate the 'KonMari Method', 'Hygge Your Home', or 'Feng Shui Your Space' you will still have to declutter your home at some point. Today's ritual is going to cover quite a lot regarding decluttering your home. This information is really important and can really help improve your home and wellness by alleviating stress and that feeling of being overwhelmed. So, let's get started.

WHAT IS DECLUTTERING?

Decluttering is removing clutter from your physical or mental space. It is discarding anything that you do not want, need or use, or getting rid of things that can make you feel stressed.

When you declutter your life, you can benefit in the following ways:

1. Have a clearer vision for yourself
2. Awaken new and positive energy
3. Be a good role model for your family
4. Boost your productivity.

1. PROMOTE PEACE AND HARMONY IN YOUR HOME

My wellness brand is all about promoting peace, harmony and wellbeing in your life. I also carry this mission statement throughout my home and surroundings. Clutter in our lives not only creates mess, but absolute chaos. By getting rid of the clutter in your home, you can discover the space and order that you seek in your life. This can bring a lot of mental clarity and a huge sense of wellbeing.

How to Maintain Harmony Whilst Decluttering

Here are some tips that may help you on your decluttering journey:

• Set aside some time each day to declutter your home, wardrobe, makeup, emails etc.

• Don't get overwhelmed by the task ahead - only do what you can do at one time and break it up into smaller parts if you need to.

• Once filtered into smaller parts, complete each small part then move onto the next.

• Avoid causing more clutter whilst you are decluttering - if you are donating things, then take them to the charity shop on the same day, do not leave things lying around.

• Get other family members to help and support you.

Stay on track and don't get distracted by other things. You can reorganise once you have decluttered.

- Have an ongoing maintenance plan. How can you keep on top of the clutter going forwards? You can sort through post as you get it rather than store it in a drawer or leaving it on a table. Deal with things right away (this includes emails too).

- Declutter by category, not by room using the KonMari Method by Marie Kondo, as we discussed earlier. It is most effective because a lot of the time, we store things in more than one place and then forget about them. By sorting through all the books in your house at once or all the clothes, you can see fully what 'sparks joy' in your life and what doesn't - you can discard what you no longer need.

- Keep only what 'sparks joy'. When you keep only the things you love, then that 'sparks joy' within you and makes you focus on only having and doing the things that make you happy. When you only have the things that make you happy in your life, you can find things easier and save both your time and your energy. Having lots of clutter of meaningless things in our homes can cause tension with family members - there can be lots of arguments and frustrations because of this. Your time is then wasted stressing about the mess and arguing about it rather than spending quality time with your family.

2. HAVE A CLEARER VISION FOR YOURSELF

If you are finding yourself making excuses as to why you can't get things done, it could be because of all the junk in your home.

The more clutter and junk that you have, the harder it is to find anything. An organised home allows you to see things clearer and find things better. You can also become more focused on your goals in life because other things are not cluttering your mind.

Here's a real-life example of how decluttering can help you:

> *Your friends have invited you out for a meal. Your closet is so full and cluttered that you can't choose what to wear, which then causes you to become very stressed and overwhelmed. You can't choose an outfit with all the clutter. You decide you have nothing to wear and then make an excuse to not go out with your friends. If everything had been neat and organised and in their proper places, this scenario would have been completely different. You would have chosen a great outfit with ease and no stress and had a great night out with your friends.*

Clutter causes your brain to go into overdrive and try to multitask, whether you want it to or not. This is because it can feel overwhelmed. Decluttering keeps you focused on what is important and what adds value to your life.

3. AWAKEN NEW AND POSITIVE ENERGY

Feng Shui is a philosophy that uses the forces of energy to allow a person to harmonise with their surroundings. Feng Shui advocates believe that this free-flowing energy (chi) generates abundance, wealth, love and health. A tidy home will make you feel calm and refreshed.

How Can Clutter Disrupt Flow in Your Life?

Clutter stops energy from flowing positively and freely. It

can cause tiredness, frustration and inactivity. Would you want to create this type of energy in your home? After decluttering, how does the new energy feel in your space? Do you feel confined or constricted in your space when it is messy? A decluttered home produces positive chi, which can help brighten your life by bringing more joy into it.

Other Ways of Boosting Chi in Your Home

Place photos of cherished memories with family and friends around your home and use natural items such as plants and flowers to decorate.

4. BE A GOOD ROLE MODEL FOR YOUR FAMILY

Through decluttering, you can be a great role model for your friends, family and children by keeping a tidy home. How can you inspire and motivate others to do the same? The answer is simply to become more organised. When people around you see your beautiful and tidy home, it may motivate them to do the same.

5. BOOST YOUR PRODUCTIVITY

When you are not organised, it takes more time for you to find what you are looking for. It also makes it harder to prioritise what needs to be done next. This can cause you to use more energy and procrastinate rather than be productive. When things are orderly, you feel in control and so your productivity increases.

Clutter is overwhelming and causes you to be unproductive and become frustrated. When you are frustrated, you are more likely to do things like surf the web, waste time on social media and not do the important things you need to do. As you go through your home, room by room, removing the clutter, you will feel more motivated to continue decluttering your home and your life. This in turn will increase your productivity levels.

TRANSFORM YOUR LIFE WITH DECLUTTERING

Where in your life can you improve your productivity? What do your current health and stress levels look like? Decluttering your kitchen can really help you to be healthier. You can clear out all the unhealthy foods and those that have gone past their sell-by date. By decluttering your kitchen, you can make your mind, body and space a healthier and happier place. By seeing healthier food in your cupboards, you are actively encouraging yourself to make better eating choices.

Decluttering allows us to have a smaller 'to do list'. Having to work around the clutter in your home makes the time to complete tasks nearly double. Less clutter means that it is easier to keep a tidy home, leaving you extra time to work on your own personal goals in life.

By getting rid of the clutter, you get rid of the stress and tension that it had on you and your family. Ever heard of the saying 'less is more'? The less clutter that is in your home, the calmer and more peaceful you feel, thus creating a wonderfully happy and clutter-free home.

It is important that you don't just declutter your home, but you declutter your digital life too.

DIGITAL DETOX

As an introvert, I find social media very overwhelming at times. For some, there is a constant need to check your phone for updates or messages, whereas for me, if it was not for my daughter, husband and business, I would not have a phone.

You are constantly being targets with marketing messages like, "You need this" and "You are not enough unless you own this" and you are literally pumped with information overload from the minute you get up to the minute you go to sleep.

I understand why there is such an increase in depression, anxiety and suicidal behaviour since social media platforms developed. When you were at school, you could get away from the bully. Now, that bully comes into your living room via your phone and there is no escape. Alternatively, through 'networking' or work emails, there is no downtime. We then end up repeating this cycle day after day.

Email marketing, text messages, spam calls, junk post – it is enough to drive anyone insane when we are connected 24/7.

It is important to take regular breaks from your social media and your phone so that you can recharge yourself! Too much downloaded information on your brain can lead to burnout, the same as when a phone needs an upgrade or shuts down entirely because of lack of memory left.

WHY HAVE A REGULAR DIGITAL DETOX?

All the technology that we surround ourselves with daily, all outputs electromagnetic fields (EMF), which with overexposure can leave some people feeling very tired, dizzy and having sensitivity to light and noise. Healing crystals can aid in deflecting some of these EMFs and lessen the effects of these devices.

What we see, eat, touch and feel is what we absorb. So, if you immerse yourself with bad news every day, you will energetically feel low, depressed and anxious. At the beginning of the Covid-19 pandemic. I had no choice but to watch the UK daily news updates which were led by the government and on for nearly an hour each day. As the minutes passed and more bad news and deaths were announced, bit by bit, I would feel my energy drain away. I understood that I had to be aware of what was going on, but I did not have to immerse myself in it. I now proactively make myself aware of my energetic drains and will quickly get a 10-minute update through the news each day and then carry on with my day. Yes, they were anxious times and, as I write this, it is still ongoing. However, me dwelling on the worry about the dire situation of our world's pandemic will not help my mental state of mind. It is awareness of your mental state that you must be very careful of in times of uncertainty and a digital detox is extremely important at these times for your own reflection.

So, learn to have a regular declutter and digital detox each day to declutter your mind, body *and* space.

This now leads us to today's *The GLOW Ritual* **for Letting Go…**

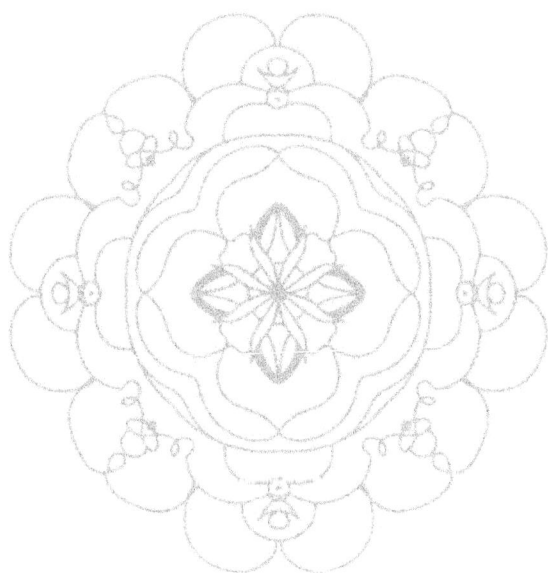

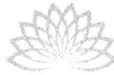

THE GLOW RITUAL
FOR LETTING GO

GRATITUDE & GET CREATIVE
Journaling Prompts

- Write down an area of the house that you would like to declutter today and how you plan to declutter it
- Write down 5 things in your life that you want to declutter to make your life happier
- Write down 5 things you are grateful for today

LIVE HOLISTICALLY
Life Lessons

- Decluttering all areas of your life is great for your wellbeing
- Having a regular digital detox is great for your mental health
- Having a tidy home can help to give you a tidy mind
- You absorb the energy you surround yourself with

ORGANISE YOUR LIFE
Get Organised

What areas of your life are making you feel drained or is using a lot of your time and energy? Today, get organised in this area. Have you got too many apps or social media accounts? What can you do to organise the digital areas of your life?

WELLNESS RITUALS
Time For Self-Care

Step away from the phone and have a digital detox day! I promise that you will feel the benefits of having a day off. Go to a spa, go for a walk, read your favourite book or even have a picnic. Observe how the time away from your phone and computer has made you feel.

I would love to see *The GLOW Ritual* you have decided to create for yourself today.

Don't forget to also tick each part of *The GLOW Ritual* off each day to support you in living your *Glowing Life Of Wellness*:

Gratitude & **G**et Creative
Live Holistically
Organise Your Life
Wellness Rituals

Share with me www.jaikooven.co.uk

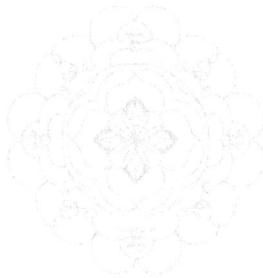

DAY 4
A RITUAL FOR A POSITIVE MONEY MINDSET

*'Working because you want to, not because
you have to is financial freedom.'*
Tony Robbins

THE RITUAL OF A POSITIVE MONEY MINDSET

You might have heard somebody say, "What is the root cause of your problem?" and this can refer to an imbalance in your Root Chakra. Your Root Chakra is what keeps you grounded and when you are out of balance, you can often feel all over the place, focus on lack, feel stuck and notice that you are scattered with your energy. So, this ritual today is all about focusing on making sure that you have enough to survive and thrive in life, rather than focusing on what you lack.

When you focus on lack, you are not being grateful for what you have, and you are not bringing more positive wealth and happiness into your life. You are a magnet for the money that you attract in your life.

MONEY MANIFESTOR

The Root Chakra is all about manifesting. For example, manifesting the money that you want and the life that you want to live. Create a plan with your money. What is the money for? What would it feel like to have that money? When you focus on lack, that is what you will bring to your life and to your wallet. Be grateful for everything that you have, keep working hard, and create a positive money mindset, then wealth and prosperity will pour into your life from all directions. For you to value money, you have to first value yourself.

Money Mindsets are about your relationship with money; your spending and saving habits, how you plan your budgets and how you were conditioned with money growing up. You would have also been influenced by the relationship that your parents had with money and how this affected your life.

SHOPAHOLIC SYNDROME

When I was younger, I was a shopaholic who spent frivolously and was completely clueless about money management. When I would go into a shop, I would find something I liked and knew that I just 'had to have it' and so the debt ball and guilt of spending continued to spiral. Those purchases also played on my self-worth. If I had the next designer bag, I would feel popular. If I bought the expensive designer perfume, it would make me feel beautiful.

However, over the years, I soon came to realise that as amazing as all of these purchases were, they did not actually make me feel better about myself in the long run. I realized that this was a huge problem and that it did not only just affect myself, but other people too.

The relationship that we, as a society, have built with materialism, self-worth and debt has caused us a huge amount of stress and worry. Having money or nice things can make you feel abundant, however lack of money or self-worth can make you feel anxious and depressed.

Money can take you wherever you want to go in life, buy you the latest designer handbag or makeup, but it could also get you into thousands of pounds' worth of debt and cause you financial worry, stress and embarrassment.

Many people do not value themselves as a person, and they do not value money, so they spend more to feel good. This feel-good feeling is always short lived as the materialistic shopping buzz wears off.

RICH GIRL, POOR GIRL

Living the rich girl, poor girl lifestyle can cause you to flip between abundance and lack in quick succession which can in turn cause a massive imbalance in your life. Through debt and a negative money mindset, you can end up in a whirlwind of mess that you do not know how to get out of. How can you attract more money into your life if you are always focusing on lack rather than enjoying what you have?

It is important to take these valuable life lessons and live and learn by your mistakes. It is never too late to change your money mindset. Nothing will change unless you change. Once you realise the error of your ways, you can decide that it is time for a 'Money Makeover'. For you to do that, you first need to go to the root of your problem –often your inner child thoughts, feelings and fears about money – and revisit all the people that have had an influence on your money mindset.

OUTSIDE INFLUENCE

The people that surround you, have a huge influence on how you are brought up with money and how you spend it. If you have friends that go shopping a lot, you may feel you want to be like them, so you may end up in debt because of that. If your family saves a lot, then you may have a fear about spending money. How do your friends and family influence your relationship with money?

Unfortunately, having money can sometimes symbolise greed and it can bring out the evil in people, and so you may have fear around becoming this way if you have money.

Building a more positive money mindset can be hard if you have not had a positive role model to show you the way. However, you can be your own role model by understanding why you are so spendthrift and can learn to change. You can uncover the insecurities within yourself that make you spend and work on your inner child healing by working through past issues with money.

REBUILDING YOUR MONEY MINDSET

Rebuilding my money mindset growing up was hard because I did not have a positive role model. This is where my entrepreneur mindset stepped in. I knew that I did not want to spend my days working for someone else for not a lot of money. I knew that I did not want to have to rely on anyone else to give me that feeling of financial freedom. I knew that it all was on me to rebuild my money mindset for a more positive future. So, with that in mind, I started to plan and build my business. Instead of spending money, I would focus on how I could positively make money and do what I love. Changing this shift in mindset allowed me to live the life I live now. A stunning home with beautiful sea views, a wonderful family, doing a job I absolutely love and living in an abundant mindset in all areas of my life. However, I always remain grounded and grateful. This allows me to feel unstoppable, and so should you.

MINI MONEY MINDSET MASTERCLASS

To create a better relationship with money:

- Spend within your means
- Track your spending
- Set up a savings account
- Don't try to impress people with frivolous spending
- Learn to value yourself with self-care and mindset work
- Learn to value and be grateful for the money in your life
- Find ways to bring abundance into your life each day
- Live with an abundant mindset

It takes guts to stand up for what you believe in and make a positive change and it takes strength to step out of the corporate box to develop something truly special for you, but I promise you that changing your money mindset will change your life. Yes, it can be hard, but the only way you can move forward is to heal yourself from your past and deal with the root of your problem.

I invite you to make those positive change today. You will not regret it.

This now leads us to *The GLOW Ritual* **for a Positive Money Mindset**…

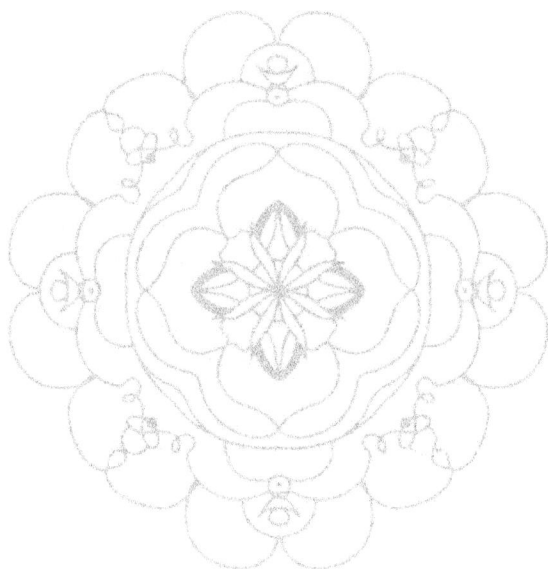

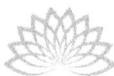

THE GLOW RITUAL
FOR A POSITIVE MONEY MINDSET

GRATITUDE & GET CREATIVE
Journaling Prompts

Write down in your journal:
- Journal about what money means to you - uncover all those thoughts, feelings and fears that you have had in the past and make note of who has influenced your money mindset
- If money were no object, what would you like to attract into your life and what would you do?
- Write down 5 things you are grateful for today

LIVE HOLISTICALLY
Life Lessons

- Discovering the roots of your money mindset can lead you to greater health, wealth and happiness in the future
- Is how you manage your money connected to your self-worth?
- Value yourself and your worth over materialistic happiness
- When you are grateful for what you have, more abundance will flow to you

ORGANISE YOUR LIFE
Get Organised

Today, spend time looking at your finances and getting them in order. Do you want to pay off a debt or save for a holiday? Organise your finances so you know exactly what is going in and out of your account and give your finances a Money Makeover.

WELLNESS RITUALS
Time for Self-Care

Create a new Money Mantra that you will repeat to yourself on a daily basis and keep in your purse or wallet. It could be something like:

"I am abundant in money and in my life. Money flows easily to me and I am grateful for everything I have."

This helps to shift your money mindset from lack to abundance each day.

I would love to see *The GLOW Ritual* you have decided to create for yourself today.

Don't forget to also tick each part of *The GLOW Ritual* off each day to support you in living your *Glowing Life Of Wellness*:

Gratitude & Get Creative
Live Holistically
Organise Your Life
Wellness Rituals

Share with me www.jaikooven.co.uk

DAY 5
A RITUAL FOR CHANGE

'The secret of change is to focus all of your energy, not on fighting the old, but on building the new.'
Socrates

ADAPTING TO CHANGE

We get so stuck in our own routines that change can be a daunting thing, whether you are adapting to being a single parent, changing jobs, or going through another big change in your life. At the time, it does feel like every inch of your life has fallen to pieces, however, if you can look at your scenario in a different light, you will see that all of these things may be happening for the greater good.

Trees shed leaves for new leaves to grow, and it works the same in your life. If you are constantly holding onto the bad things in your life, you cannot let good new things come in. So, adapt to change, embrace it with all your heart, and you never know where it could take you.

LIVING IN LOCKDOWN

I had heard of the Coronavirus Pandemic whilst I was in Hong Kong. At the time, my mum and I saw lots of people with masks on and we even wore them ourselves. Yet, we never realized at the time how much of an impact that terrible virus would then have on the world once we got back home. One minute, life was completely normal in the UK then, all of a sudden, it changed overnight. Luckily, we were not carriers of the virus, and we did not get it on our travels.

However, within a few weeks of our return, there were daily news reports of rapidly increasing deaths in the UK. This virus had now spread pretty much worldwide. In March 2020, life completely changed for everyone in the UK; businesses closed down, people lost their jobs, schools shut, and UK residents were told to 'stay at home'. Our freedom was taken away from us as the virus swept the world, and all social contact with anyone outside of our own home became illegal.

For somebody that had recovered from PTSD, I started feeling more and more anxious day by day as I became a prisoner in my own home. Nobody knew at that time that the lockdown situation would change our world in such a big way. Even as I write this in May 2021, we are still in a partial lockdown with some restaurants only just opening indoors and a new Indian variant sweeping our country. We have gone over a year without hugs from members of our family because the virus is highly contagious, and we are all currently waiting to be vaccinated.

It has been a whirlwind since we were made aware of this life-threatening virus and told by the UK government to adapt to 'the new normal' and 'stay at home'. I could feel myself starting to get those familiar feelings of panic that I used to get with PTSD. That feeling of being trapped and isolated with nowhere to go.

One feeling I identified was the feeling of being helpless and not being able to actually control the situation that I was in. For a few days during the first lockdown when everything shut, including schools, I was terrified and anxious and would spend most of my days watching the news whilst more and more bad news unfolded.

I soon found that this habit was causing me more anxiety, and I could actually control what I was exposing myself to. I decided to control what I could and stop trying to control what I couldn't. The next day, I limited the news on the TV to only the daily updates. Throughout the day, I would switch the TV off and listen to music, home school my daughter, play in the garden, make candles, study towards some more holistic qualifications and work on my business. I also channelled my energy into writing this book during this period.

I was not in control of the Coronavirus Pandemic, but I was in control of my own health and wellbeing and helping clients with theirs.

So, as always, I went back to the roots of why I created *The GLOW Ritual* and applied it to my life. I decided to be proactive rather than reactive to the situation. I would write my daily lists of things that would make me feel good and make a difference to my life and started to do *The GLOW Ritual* every day.

At a very distressing time such as this, where the whole world is changing so rapidly, it is easy to get depressed and you can just want to give up. However, I have always been a fighter and no matter what, I decided I would do everything I could to make the most of this time at home and being in this lockdown situation. I practiced gratitude and was grateful that my dear late stepdad did not have to suffer during this pandemic, or he would have died alone without the care and attention that he needed – or worse still, he could have died from the virus.

When I think about the isolation or I worry about getting the virus myself, I channel my worries into what I can control. I can make myself a healthy smoothie or a hot lemon drink. I can meditate, practice yoga or write in my journal. I can keep hygienic and keep a clean home.

Another thing I did during lockdown, was spend time with my daughter doing crafts, watching films and going for walks. I spent daily time in meditation, journaling and doing exercise. Every day, I would make sure that my positivity cup was filled. That's not to say that I did not worry sometimes, but I did not let the worry take over my mind. As soon as I felt the worry build up, I would say to myself, "What can I do to make myself better?" or "Can I change this?" I could not physically stop Coronavirus from spreading (apart from playing my part in being hygienic), but at this unpredictable time, I could take much needed time for my own self-care, making my home a sanctuary and getting organised with my business.

LEARNING TO PAUSE

I believe that life gives you lessons and living through three national lockdowns taught me so much about myself. Instead of being a hamster on an endless wheel to nowhere, I learnt the power to pause and be still. I learnt to find contentment with what I had around me and not to seek my happiness in materialistic things and spontaneous shopping hauls. I learned to quieten my mind, shifting from 'doing' to 'just being', and I learnt the immense healing power of embodying the beauty of Yin Yoga – be still and release. I talk a lot more about Yin Yoga further on in my book and I am so grateful to have this in my life. At a time when the world was and still is chaotic, I could find a calm sanctuary within myself.

As you can see, you can rewrite your story whenever you wish. When you look for the lessons that traumas in your life teach you, you grow spiritually stronger and more resilient to outside conditions when they attempt to shake you. When you are rooted to the ground, you can remain unshakeable.

DON'T DWELL ON THE PAST. LEARN FROM THE LESSONS & BUILD A BETTER FUTURE.

Changes will always happen but, it is how we adapt to those changes in a positive way that helps us get through times of struggle and unease.

This now leads us to ***The GLOW Ritual* for Change…**

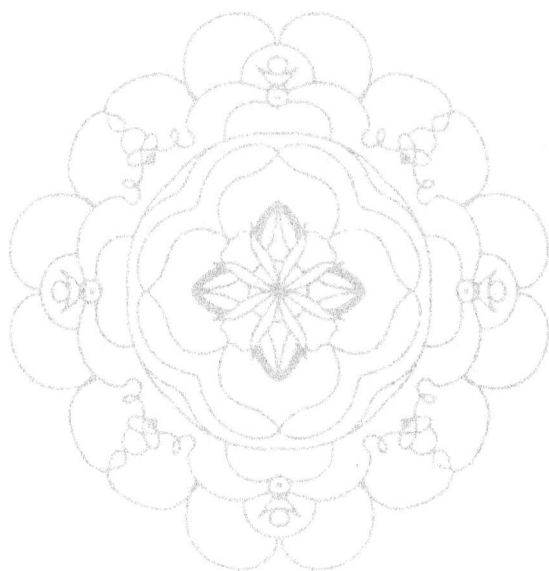

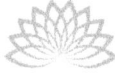

THE GLOW RITUAL
FOR CHANGE

GRATITUDE & GET CREATIVE
Journaling Prompts

Today, write in your journal:

- What would you like to change in your life?
- How do you plan to make those changes?
- How would it make you feel?
- Write down 5 things you are grateful for today

LIVE HOLISTICALLY
Life Lessons

- Learning to have time to pause and reflect is a great way for you to assess your next path
- Change is always a good thing for our personal growth
- Looking after your mental health will help to keep you grounded during times of change

ORGANISE YOUR LIFE
Get Organised

Change is inevitable and it is something that you need to embrace from time to time so you can move forward in a positive way. Today, incorporate a positive change into your life, such as changing your diet, or switching to a natural skincare range and get organised so you can easily do it as a daily habit.

WELLNESS RITUALS
Time For Self-Care

Do a meditation that can help you in adapting to change. Light a candle and spend time reflecting on the results you want from the changes you are about to make.

I would love to see *The GLOW Ritual* you have decided to create for yourself today.

Don't forget to also tick each part of *The GLOW Ritual* off each day to support you in living your *Glowing Life Of Wellness*:

Gratitude & **G**et Creative
Live Holistically
Organise Your Life
Wellness Rituals

Share with me www.jaikooven.co.uk

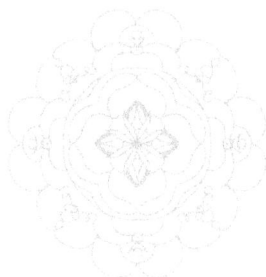

ROOT CHAKRA RITUALS

In this chapter, we covered:

- *The GLOW Ritual* for Grounding
- *The GLOW Ritual* for Strength
- *The GLOW Ritual* for Change
- *The GLOW Ritual* for Letting Go
- *The GLOW Ritual* for a Positive Money Mindset

This chapter describes the building blocks for your new foundation. We covered how to adapt to change to establish good routines, and how to be grateful for everything that you have so you can change your mindset and allow more positive things to flow into your life. You also learned how to get to the root of the problem so you could learn how to let go.

THE ROOT CHAKRA

In this section we covered all information about the Root Chakra. The Root Chakra helps us with our strength and grounding.

When you are out of balance in the Root Chakra, you can feel scattered, stuck, and have a negative money mindset.

The Root Chakra is about feeling safe and secure in your environment, as well as emotionally.

CRYSTALS FOR THE ROOT CHAKRA:

Red Jasper

Red Jasper is the overall crystal balancer for this Chakra as it is the supreme nurturer and stone of endurance.

Moss Agate

Moss Agate is known as the 'stabilizer stone'. It helps with supportive growth. It has loving Earth energy to assist you steadily enduring anything that life throws at you. It gives you the confidence of Mother Earth as you concentrate and focus on attracting financial prosperity and business success.

Blue Lace Agate

One of my favourite crystals is Blue Lace Agate which is a variety of chalcedony. Not only does it look beautiful, but it will also give you a wonderful feeling of calm and help guide you back to happiness.

Citrine

Keep Citrine in your wallet or purse and in your office as this attracts wealth and abundance.

ESSENTIAL OILS FOR THE ROOT CHAKRA

Use an essential oil diffuser to surround yourself with a choice of one of these scents or create your own uplifting mixture.

PLEASE SEEK MEDICAL OR PROFESSIONAL ADVICE IF YOU ARE PREGNANT OR HAVE A MEDICAL CONDITION.

Lemon is uplifting and enhances a positive mood.

Ginger Root is energising and grounding.

Peppermint prevents fatigue and improves exercise performance.

Pine provides a boost of energy levels.

Ylang ylang reduces depression and boosts your mood.

REFLECTION

When you look at your current life now, what could you change for a more positive life? What routines could you establish that would help you to achieve your goals and live a life you love?

POSITIVE CHANGE

Write down in your journal your answers to the above questions and, as of today, add in a section to your journal to write down three things you are grateful for each and every day.

Well done on completing your first chapter on the Root Chakra.

What did you enjoy the most about this chapter? Let me know at www.jaikooven.co.uk and don't forget to share with me your daily mini rituals too.

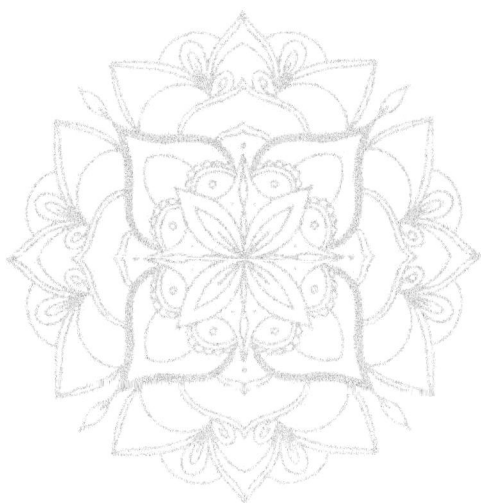

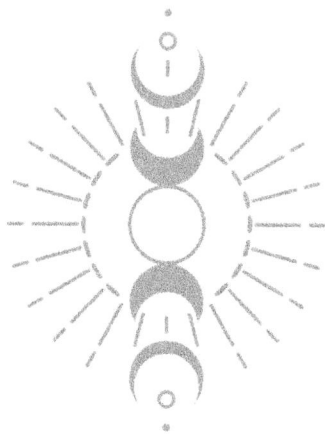

Glow with the Flow

❀

CHAPTER

Two

SACRAL CHAKRA

WHAT IS THE SACRAL CHAKRA?

The Sacral Chakra (aka *Svadhisthana*) is the Chakra of Creativity and Freedom. This Chakra is responsible for passion, creativity, intimacy, joy and sexuality. Having balance in this Chakra allows us to improve our relationships with ourselves and others. As a creative, this is one of my favourite Chakras. This Chakra also carries with it the power of partnership, how we relate to others and our creative exploration in our lives, sexuality and relationships. The Sacral Chakra focuses on how you interact and create the world around you. It also encourages you to create your own personal identity and your external world through your creative freedom and choices. A person who has strong Sacral Chakra energy can survive physically and financially on their own and bond with others to form harmonious friendships. This Chakra also focuses on our pleasures in life, whether that be sexual pleasures or doing things we find pleasure in.

The Sacral Chakra is all about discovering and utilizing your talents and expressing yourself through your creativity. It teaches us that every relationship we create has a purpose. The Sacral Chakra acts as the 'birth canal' of what we want in life. It is the manifestation womb where we can birth the life we really want and create things we only ever dreamed of. It gives us the great feeling of being alive and creating a life that we desire.

WHERE IS THE SACRAL CHAKRA LOCATED?

The Sacral Chakra is located just above the pubic bone.

WHAT COLOUR IS THE SACRAL CHAKRA?

Orange.

HOW WILL I FEEL IF THIS CHAKRA IS BALANCED?

- You will radiate warmth, generosity and confidence

- You will feel connected and grounded

- You will feel energized by your creative flow

- You can easily express yourself artistically

- Your body feels energetic, with a healthy libido and sensual life

- Your spirit feels compassionate, forgiving and joyful

- You will feel connected to your passion

HOW MIGHT I FEEL IF I AM OUT OF BALANCE?

- You may feel overwhelmed and depressed

- You may have emotional instability

- You may have loss of your creativity

- You may have addictive behaviours

- You may have low self-confidence

- You may suffer from depression and fear, feel withdrawn and in pain

- You may have a hormone imbalance, develop addictions and have a habit of indulging in things that are not good for you

- In your spirit you may feel resentful, be controlling, guilty and hold jealousy towards others

SELF-LOVE WAYS TO GET BACK IN BALANCE

- Wear orange or eat orange foods which are healthy e.g. mangoes, melon, pumpkin

- Do a Sacral Chakra Yoga Class through YouTube or through my membership programme

- Get your feelings out on paper to shift your block and allow for creative flow

DAY 6
A RITUAL FOR HEALING YOUR INNER CHILD

*'Every child is an artist. The problem is how to remain
an artist once he grows up.'*
Pablo Picasso

THE HOME OF YOUR INNER CHILD

The Sacral Chakra is the home of your inner child – that part of you that has been rejected, denied, neglected and abandoned, and the part of us that we try our best to hide. All of us have an inner child within ourselves that represents sensitivity, playfulness, joy, awe, wonder and innocence.

The prominent psychological thinker Sigmund Freud suggested that mental difficulties and our most destructive behaviours experienced by adults are related to trauma experienced by the inner child. He continues to explain that our lack of understanding, our inner child, is what can cause relationship difficulties, emotional problems and behavioural problems in the future. Another way of framing this is that we are dissociated from our inner child as we get older. Due to this dissociation, it can cause us to become 'stuck' in our psychological development. We may have grown up biologically, but out development psychologically has not caught up.

It does not help in society when we are told to 'grow up', 'stop being sensitive' or to 'just move on'. As an adult, our playfulness, joy, innocence, wonder and sensitivity are slowly stripped away as we are conditioned into adult life. We are told to bury our emotions as we grow into adulthood and because of this our inner child is neglected, abandoned, denied and rejected.

HOW DOES YOUR INNER CHILD AFFECT YOUR ADULT LIFE?

I understand first-hand how my inner child has affected me in my later life. My experience of living in a council house next to a drug dealer and having his unconscious clients passed out on my doorstep caused me a lot of damage in my adult life. It led me to have an unhealthy relationship with my home as a child and as an adult. When I was younger, I was so ashamed of my home, I would make excuses not to have friends over. As I grew older, my home became my everything and it is really important to me that I feel safe and that it is orderly and calm.

It is a standard I have that my home should look a certain way and I still cannot stand mess and disorder in my home, even though I have healed my inner child wounds. However, I am a lot better than I was before.

Before, if there was mess in my home, I would make excuses not to have friends over or I would drive myself to an anxiety attack, trying to make my home feel welcome to them by frantically tidying up. I love Feng Shui and I believe every home has a heartbeat and energy to it. If my house is ever messy, I feel the negative energy immediately. I feel oppressed, trapped, anxious, sad, unmotivated and embarrassed. As soon as the house is tidy again, that energy lifts and the tidiness clears the air and I feel I can breathe again. I am proud of my home, and I feel I can open it up to my friends and family now which I really struggled with when I was younger. I did not realise until a few years ago, how much my inner child influenced my behaviours as an adult. My issues with my home as a child kept me feeling helpless to change my circumstances at the time and when I have a messy home or DIY going on, these feelings would rear their ugly head again.

I now understand how to heal these feelings and my emotions regarding my home, and I feel a lot more in control. I know how to manage my home to make it a lovely clean space as well as it still feeling homely.

CHILDHOOD VS ADULTHOOD

Childhood fears, traumas, hurt and anger are also part of our inner child personality. When we 'grow up' as adults, we think because we are older that our childhood issues are behind us, and we may be harsh on our childhood selves because of our innocence and sensitivity.

Denying your inner child's needs does not make them go away as we are then controlled by them in later life, and this can happen unconsciously. Despite our best efforts as an adult, we are not able to make good choices and self-direct our own lives. Instead, our thoughts, feelings and actions are guided by the hurt, wounded, angry and vulnerable inner child within us. It is like having a 6-year-old child in a 35-year-old body. Therefore, many psychologists believe that bad decisions can be made in adult life along with experiencing mental and emotional difficulties and poor relationships. It is the unrecognized inner child within us that is playing havoc with our adult brain and reliving our childhood as an adult over and over again.

THE INNER CHILD TRAUMA

As a result of trauma from our childhood, psychologists believe that our psychological growth becomes suppressed and stunted.

There are many traumas which you may have experienced as a child that will still affect you now as an adult. These include:

- Neglect, being ignored or disrespected
- Abuse of any kind – sexual, emotional, mental
- Abandonment
- Tragic events
- Lack of approval, affirmation or support
- Growing up without emotional boundaries

As we grow older, we create a strong barrier between ourselves and the world to help us deal with trauma as an adult. We put this mask on to protect ourselves from further hurt, rather than heal our emotional wounds. However, suppression of any kind causes a lot of damage, especially when you are suppressing your inner child emotions.

The trauma experienced as a child can have a significant negative impact on your adult life, especially the feeling of self-worth and self-confidence. As a child, you may have been told you were never good enough or that you would always fail or that starting your own business was too risky. These words echo in your adult brain and then your self-belief falls at the wayside whilst you just 'settle' in a secure job that makes you unhappy rather than realise your own true potential.

These negative words spoken by parents, friends or family will have stuck with you in later life which will lead you to feeling like:

- You are not good enough
- You are not worthy
- You will never make it in life

- You are a nobody
- Why would people want to be your friend?
- You will not be a success

These adult thoughts become our feelings, which will in turn cause us to behave and live our lives in a certain way. You suppress the 'real you' because you are too scared to be your true self and are afraid of being exposed as a failure. Therefore, many wannabe entrepreneurs never try to make their dreams come true. The fear of failure or judgement is so great that they never heal their inner child and move on to achieving their goals in life.

Not only does this negativity affect our thoughts about ourselves, but it also affects how we see the world, our life and the people around us. We can pick up negative beliefs about our society and life. These may include:

- I cannot trust anyone
- Everyone is better than me
- I am an imposter
- People just use me for money
- I will never get married because it will end in divorce
- I am not worthy of love

I absolutely love reading and learning, and this was built into me at a young age. I recently read *Best Self – Be You, Only Better* by life coach Mike Bayer who talks briefly about the effects of inner child trauma. He writes:

Children are blank slates, and in the early years, our parents and others write on those slates for us. But it is important to know our original stories nonetheless, so that we can be aware of whether we are expressing ourselves as adults in a way that aligns with who we truly are and, more important, to understand if any negative aspects of our origin story might be affecting our current behaviour in some fashion ...

Life happens around us and through our experiences, we define who we are or who we believe we are.

You cannot change your childhood, but you can change your future. So, create new thoughts and beliefs about your situation as an adult. See how much better and lighter it makes you feel when you let go of your childhood baggage.

This now leads us to *The GLOW Ritual* **for Healing Your Inner Child**…

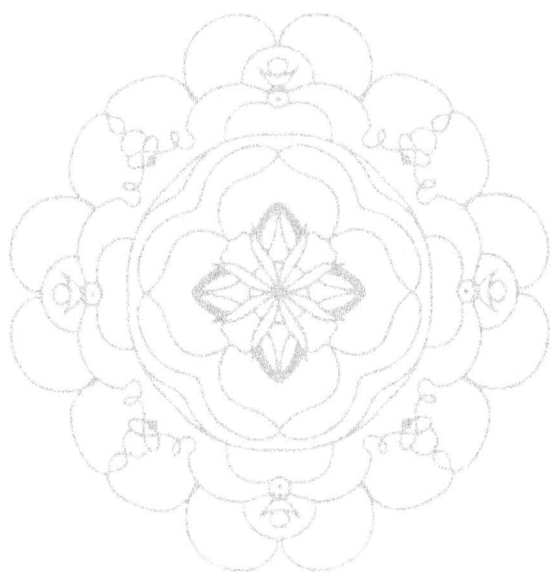

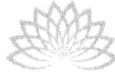

THE GLOW RITUAL
FOR HEALING YOUR INNER CHILD

GRATITUDE & GET CREATIVE
Journaling Prompts

Today, write in your journal:

- What areas in your life need inner child healing?
- What trauma did you go through to feel or act this way?
- How can you respond differently in your adult life to get the results you want?
- Write down 5 things you are grateful for today

LIVE HOLISTICALLY
Life Lessons

- Understand how your childhood traumas affect your adult life
- Identify areas of your life that need healing
- Make positive changes moving forwards

ORGANISE YOUR LIFE
Get Organised

Today, you are going to identify areas in your life that need inner child healing. Observe negative habits that you have carried with you since childhood and break the cycle by changing that habit to something that the adult version of you would do.

WELLNESS RITUALS
Time For Self-Care

Now you have identified areas of your life that need healing today, make time to nurture yourself and your space. What would make you feel amazing today? An indulgent bath with beautiful aromas, time in the garden painting your nails or even a herbal tea to give you a comforting hug in a mug.

I would love to see *The GLOW Ritual* you have decided to create for yourself today.

Don't forget to also tick each part of *The GLOW Ritual* off each day to support you in living your *Glowing Life Of Wellness*:

Gratitude & **G**et Creative
Live Holistically
Organise Your Life
Wellness Rituals

Share with me www.jaikooven.co.uk

DAY 7
A RITUAL FOR NEW BEGINNINGS

'I never dreamed about success. I worked for it.'
Estee Lauder

BELIEVING IN YOURSELF

Low confidence and poor self-esteem are very common in this modern world, so you are never alone if you feel this way.

For years, I always felt like I was trying to hide myself from the world. For some reason, maybe because I am quite introverted, I just wanted to be invisible. I hated having my picture taken and, whenever I knew there was a video chat going on, I would literally run and hide. It made me feel exposed in my own home and very unsettled. I also absolutely hated social media.

Then in 2020, through personal growth, I turned a corner. I realized that I had spent all these years running, hiding and trying to be invisible, but why? What did I have to hide? Why did I want to be invisible?

There is a famous quote that I absolutely love which sums up how I live my life:

> *"And one day she discovered that she was*
> *fierce and strong, and full of fire, and that not*
> *even she could hold herself back because her*
> *passion burned brighter than her fears."*
> *Mark Anthony*

That was exactly how I felt! One day, I literally 'woke up' both spiritually and mentally and just knew that I am here to help bring a positive message to the world and despite my fears, my passion to help others overcame every fear I had of being visible and seen. I slowly learnt that if I did not believe in myself, then how can anyone ever believe in me?

There are many times in life where you can run and hide or stand up and face your fears. Facing your fears allows you to grow as a person, build on your strengths and weaknesses and stand up and be proud of the person that you have become.

Every person in the world started somewhere. We have all lacked confidence at certain points in our lives and questioned who we are or who we should be.

We have all had failures and successes and have all experienced rejection a multiple number of times. Rejection should never be the reason why you stop what you are passionate about and quit. Rejection should be the thing that spurs you on to work harder or change your strategy to achieve your success. Even if one person may not like what you are doing, another person will.

The most influential people are the people that stand up for what they believe in, stand true to who they are and don't let anyone dull the light that they bring to this world.

This now leads us to *The GLOW Ritual* for New Beginnings...

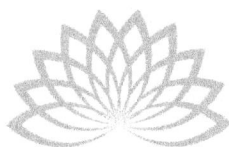

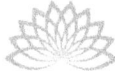

THE GLOW RITUAL
FOR NEW BEGINNINGS

GRATITUDE & GET CREATIVE
Journaling Prompts

Today, write in your journal:

- What areas are you lacking in confidence? What was your earliest memory which has caused you to have this belief?
- How can you change your mindset going forwards?
- What are the benefits of you believing in yourself? How will your life be different?
- Write down 5 things you are grateful for today

LIVE HOLISTICALLY
Life Lessons

- Learn to believe in yourself and your talents to discover a whole world of possibility
- Learn to be visible and stand tall and proud of your achievements
- Rejection should not make you stop what you are passionate about - it should spur you to change your strategy to achieve your success

ORGANISE YOUR LIFE
Get Organised

Today you will have a confidence boost day, by spending a few hours (or the day) working on a project that you always wanted to do. Identify how this makes you feel and the confidence that you have gained by doing something you always wanted to do.

WELLNESS RITUALS
Time For Self-Care

Today, spend time in reflection of how you want your new beginning to start. What did you not like about your old way of living and what new energy would you like to bring into your life now?

Play some music that makes you feel uplifted as you write in your journal and plan your new life. Finish with a relaxing bathing ritual to cleanse your mind, body and soul to reveal a new and revitalized you.

I would love to see **The GLOW Ritual** you have decided to create for yourself today.

Don't forget to also tick each part of **The GLOW Ritual** off each day to support you in living your **Glowing Life Of Wellness**:

Gratitude & Get Creative
Live Holistically
Organise Your Life
Wellness Rituals

Share with me www.jaikooven.co.uk

DAY 8
A RITUAL FOR EMPOWERMENT

'It is not in the stars to hold
our destiny but ourselves.'
Shakespeare

FEELING EMPOWERED

I have always had an entrepreneurial mindset, been open-minded to change, loved learning new things and have been very ambitious from a young age.

I have always had an ambitious fire that burned within me and never went away. I always knew that I was not meant to work for others and that I would eventually find my own path.

When I discovered the world of holistic wellness, personal development and spirituality 15 years ago, it really changed my life and how I see the world. I was inspired by learning positive rituals to help me grow as a person. I would spend hours studying the habits and routines that made people successful in life and in their wellbeing.

One of the first self-help books I ever read has always stuck in my head as I must have read it a million times. It's called *The Miracle Morning* by Hal Elrod and talks about the benefits of a good morning routine and getting up early to improve all areas of your life and your productivity. When I started to follow Hal's advice, incredible things started to happen. I had more energy, felt more positive, was healthier and fitter and achieved so much in the mornings before the whole world had woken up.

Since then, I have spent years mastering my daily rituals in order to create a successful and meaningful life.

RITUALS FOR AMBITIOUS WOMEN

When I read *Daily Rituals Women at Work* by Mason Currey, it looked at the rituals of very influential women in this world, from Nina Simone to Coco Chanel. It looked at their day-to-day lives and their incredible creative minds that contributed to them becoming great role models for women all over the world. It was then that I was intrigued to discover what takes these ordinary women and makes them extraordinary. I was inspired to be like them.

This is what focused my mindset as an ambitious woman, and I knew that my mission was to empower other women to achieve great things in their lives and to not just settle for second best.

As busy modern women, we are constantly juggling our various roles in life. Especially if, and when, we become mothers – our roles change completely. We often go from career women to full-time parent for our precious babies. As our babies grow, we then have to rediscover ourselves, our careers and prove ourselves to the world, whilst juggling motherhood, being a wife, cleaner, and cook.

There is huge demand on our time and, therefore, many of us forget our ambition out of pure exhaustion of trying to be everything to everyone. Many of us forget our goals in life and just settle for a simpler way of living with less complications so it can fit around childcare. This is fine for many that want that life, but for the ambitious career women, we need something else. You should never have to 'settle' in life. Your babies will grow older and will have their own lives and you are still an individual with dreams that you can achieve even as a parent.

If you want something in life, you will do anything to achieve that goal. There are always daily obstacles standing in your way and different people and things demanding our attention. You can have two women, with the same lifestyle, with the same amount of demands in life and yet, they will both have different results. Why is that? The difference is that one woman will have ambition, determination, creativity and motivation and have the fire within them that no matter what, they will never give up. They will make sacrifices daily to achieve their goals as they know there is no other option. Whilst the other woman will often be waiting for the perfect opportunity or for something to fall on their lap. Success does not just happen – you must make it happen and sometimes you may need to graft for years and years before success finally comes to you.

We are all guilty of sometimes having a 'Netflix and chill night'. However, for the woman that wants to build her empire or build a better lifestyle, there needs to be an element of self-discipline to get what you want. It never feels like a sacrifice when you are learning and building a strategy for your own self-improvement.

It is all about balance whilst still making space for your downtime. However, if I am on a deadline for an article or manuscript submission then I understand that in order for me to achieve anything in life, I have to put in the effort in order to get the results that I require. I still get to pick my daughter up from school and drop her off in the mornings, and I still deal with household responsibilities and attend school plays. I have created a career around a life that I want to lead, where there is no sacrifice for living a life you absolutely love whilst being of service to others.

My inner fire tells me that I no longer want to play small in life and that I can achieve everything I set out to do, and you can too. I have worked with many women in the past that tell me that they 'do not have time' and I tell them that you make the time for the things that matter to you! So, if you don't want to be stuck in a 9-5 job that you hate, then you don't have to. You can do and be anything you want in life. It takes motivation and discipline, but you can do it and don't let anything stand in your way, not even fear of failure.

DON'T BE AFRAID TO FAIL

The only failure in life is not to try in the first place. I see failure as an opportunity to learn and grow, see where I went wrong, learn the life lessons, and find a new way forward. The one thing that I do not fear is failure because I will always keep trying, and I know with certainty that one day something will just click.

> *"Whenever I'm faced with a difficult decision,*
> *I ask myself: What would I do if I weren't*
> *afraid of making a mistake, feeling rejected,*
> *looking foolish, or being alone?*
> *I know for sure that when you remove fear, the*
> *answer you've been searching for comes into*
> *focus."*
> *Oprah Winfrey*

FEEL EMPOWERED TO KEEP GOING

I can't explain what spurs me on. Maybe it's because when I was 12, I had a brain tumour and still, to this day, there is a small part of the tumour still in my brain. When you are faced with death at a very young age and the possibility that the brain tumour could grow again, even now, it makes you look at life differently.

For me, there is no tomorrow – there is only today. I know 100% that if I keep working and trying new things, one day something will just click, and I will get my desired result. I never know where my creative ideas will take me; I just follow my intuition with renewed courage to keep moving forwards. For me, that is the only option as I will never give up. Like when you play a video game, you fail many times, but you dust yourself off, learn a new strategy and start again. Even as I write *The GLOW Ritual*, I am currently 47,112 words into a 60,000 book and boy has it been an emotional ride, but it has been worth it! At times it has felt like a marathon, but now I am nearing completion, it is a sprint towards the end.

As I was writing *The GLOW Ritual* and got to 45,000 words, my intuition was telling me that something was not working. I could not get into the flow of writing. So, at this stage, I restructured my whole book to fit in with what I envisaged I wanted *The GLOW Ritual* to represent.

It just goes to show that it is never too late to adapt or start again. Do not be afraid to adapt things in your life if you need to. Don't be afraid to change your mind. Change offers new adventures and opportunity to learn and grow. You will never fail if you always try your best.

You can create any life you want, and we are all artists of our own lives. When will you start creating your masterpiece?

This now leads us to *The GLOW Ritual* **for Empowerment**...

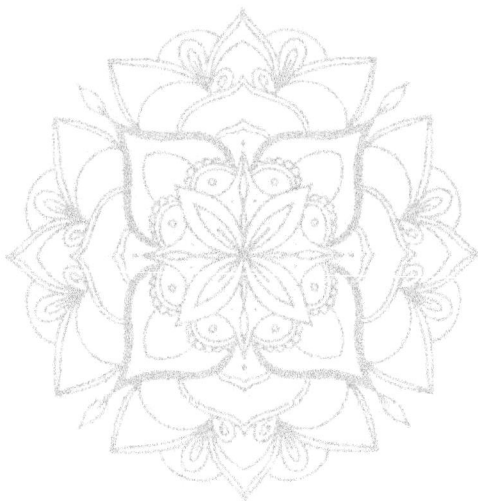

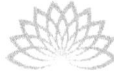

THE GLOW RITUAL
FOR EMPOWERMENT

GRATITUDE & GET CREATIVE
Journaling Prompts

Today, write in your journal:

- What areas are you lacking confidence in? What was your earliest memory which has caused you to have this belief?
- How can you change your mindset going forwards?
- What are the benefits of believing in yourself? How will your life be different?
- What are 5 things that you are grateful for today?

LIVE HOLISTICALLY
Life Lessons

- You can always change your mind - change offers new adventures and opportunities
- Create daily rituals to keep you motivated and empowered
- Don't be afraid to fail

ORGANISE YOUR LIFE
Get Organised

Today, identify a course that you would like to take to learn something new that would empower you to pursue your goals. If you can't afford to do a course right now, spend some time doing research on your chosen topic that will support you in building your confidence.

WELLNESS RITUALS
Time For Self-Care

Today, start your day 30-minutes earlier with gratitude. As you are getting dressed, be grateful for the person that you are. Acknowledge your good qualities but also areas that you can improve. Embrace your empowerment by spending time doing a 10-minute yoga flow for empowerment or self-confidence.

I would love to see *The GLOW Ritual* you have decided to create for yourself today.

Don't forget to also tick each part of *The GLOW Ritual* off each day to support you in living your *Glowing Life Of Wellness*:

Gratitude & **G**et Creative
Live Holistically
Organise Your Life
Wellness Rituals

Share with me www.jaikooven.co.uk

DAY 9
A RITUAL FOR CREATIVE FLOW

*'Those who flow as life flows know
they need no other force.'*
Lao Tzu

FINDING YOUR FLOW & CREATE YOUR INNER GLOW

The GLOW Ritual is all about creating an inner glow through living a **Glowing Life Of Wellness**, embracing holistic living and finding your creativity through journaling and channelling your creativity. 'A Ritual for Creative Flow' means to understand the feelings you get when everything feels aligned and just flows easily. You know in your heart that you are doing something you absolutely love which feeds your soul. This could be a creative business or just doing your favourite hobby. Whatever it is, it makes you glow from the inside out and time just stands still when you are doing it. This is how I feel as I write this book, when I mentor my clients and when I create content for my business. I get lost in a creative world where I feel like anything is possible. Doing a career that I absolutely love allows me to achieve that flow state each day as I live and breathe holistic living and creativity. I love what I do, and I want to help you to learn how to do the same.

Although, it has not always been this way for me. From the age of three, I always remember making things with my late grandmother and my mum. We were a very creative family and the things we made were endless; decorated eggs, handmade cards, crochet, knitting, painting, jewellery, etc. We would make art out of anything and our world was literally our canvas to create something beautiful. However, even though I could create things, I could not draw to save my life! I loved the creative process of making things with my family and something really sparked in me from such a young age.

As I got older, my creativity blossomed into writing, and I qualified in London as a journalist. I worked for an amazing magazine publishing company and loved every minute of it. Then I needed to relocate, so I had to find a new job. As part of my journalism studies, I studied law, so I decided to work for a law firm. Wow, what a change to my creative life! The money was great; however, I was miserable and the people I worked with were miserable too. I spent my days praying that lunch would come around, so I could be creative and make things. To the point where, on my lunchbreaks, I created my own handmade jewellery business, created a jewellery website and got featured on the front page of a wedding magazine!

My desk space was uninspiring and oppressive. The rooms of the office were unmotivating, depressing and I just knew that I was not here on this Earth to be a corporate robot. I often thought, "When I die, I will be in a box, but I certainly don't want to work in one until that happens!" This is when the fire inside me decided to pursue what I loved and live a life of flow every day.

As, a part of my job as an author and international holistic expert, I find the subject of the Flow State fascinating. Learning to understand the Flow State is important as it enables you to understand how your mind works and what makes you feel holistically whole.

'Getting into the flow' or 'Flow State' is one of my favourite things to do and feel. As you can see, you can 'find your flow' in many different things. For me, it was making jewellery, being creative, writing, doing a career I love and practicing yoga.

WHAT IS FLOW STATE?

A Flow State is when you are completely and utterly immersed in what you are doing. Time stands still and all that matters is what you are doing at that present time. There is no worry about judgement or failure. I achieve Flow State when I do yoga or use my creative energy to create something beautiful, like this book. Energetically, Flow State makes you feel great, and you can feel on top of the world doing what you love. You can also achieve a Flow State when you cook, when you are cleaning, doing a hobby, reading or out in nature, to name a few. It does not matter what it is that gets you into a Flow State if it makes you feel good. So, let's discover how to master your own Flow State…

THE PSYCHOLOGY OF POSITIVITY AND FLOW

Positive Psychology has a huge focus on *Eudaimonia. Eudaimonia* is a term used for living a 'good life' or 'flourishing life'. It is encouraged that you live a fulfilling life, focused on the things you love that bring great joy to your life. We are all unique and individual, therefore, a happy life looks different for everyone in the world. As Marie Kondo would say "Do what sparks joy."

Positive Psychology compliments traditional psychological approaches in encouraging you to behave in a positive way which aids your development. Using Positive Psychology, you are able to achieve a life that you desire where you feel fulfilled and inspired to be the best version of you.

Positive self-esteem and self-image can help you redirect your positivity to achieve a life of your dreams, with nothing holding you back. Positive Psychology can help you be driven by your thoughts of the future rather than be held back by the past. However, purely focusing on the future can have a negative effect as it can tend to discourage you if your goals feel too far away. Therefore, positive psychologists promote seeing positive experiences in the current moment, rather than always focusing on the future. As a result, Positive Psychology can help you have a mental shift to see the future with optimism because you are always living in the moment and enjoying each day.

THE THREE LEVELS OF POSITIVE PSYCHOLOGY

We all look at the world differently and react individually to various situations that face us. Many years ago, when I first started studying Cognitive Behavioural Therapy (CBT), this concept amazed me. You could have three individuals each faced with the same scenario and each person would have a unique outcome based on their thoughts, feelings and actions towards that scenario.

Here's an example where there are three people that work at the same job. The company is starting to expand and there are a lot of changes going on:

Person 1 has a negative response to the changes. They do not like change so moan to family, friends and colleagues. This affects their focus on work and then their results, which over time leads to them getting the sack. People also find them annoying because they moan all the time and so they do not have many friends.

Person 2 accepts the changes and is open minded to new things. They are comfortable and happy with their job so just carry on as normal, and their job and circumstances stay the same.

Person 3 sees the changes as a huge opportunity to get noticed and promoted in their work. They embrace the changes and new training with positivity, and this results in them getting a promotion. People around Person 3 feel inspired by the energy they give off and because of this, they have a lot of friends.

It is interesting when you see this same scenario carried out, but with three very different outcomes based on the power of our mind.

MORE ABOUT FLOW STATE

As I explained earlier, Flow State is where you are so focused on your current task that you go into your own world. You are barely aware of your current surroundings because you are so involved in what you are doing. Another example of Flow State is when I am reading a book. I get so immersed in all the characters and the location of the story, that I forget that I just boiled the kettle until it clicks off. The reason for this is because my brain dedicates a huge amount of its processing power to the task that I am currently doing. It barely registers the sensory information that it is being given.

THE ELEMENTS OF FLOW STATE

Even though what we are doing to experience a Flow State differs from person to person, the experience of Flow State is the same for everyone. The experience would be exactly the same for somebody making jewellery as it would be for someone building a motorbike.

Our feelings of wellbeing and enjoyment are usually based on doing goal-orientated activities with a set of rules attached to them. However, to feel fulfilled in these activities, there has to be a balance between the skills you have and the challenges the activity poses to your skill set. The challenge of the activity will influence how much you will enjoy the activity.

When you are in Flow State, you are laser focused on the task in hand. There is no divide between you and your task as you merge into oneness where time stands still, and you are lost in a different world. However, if you lose your concentration or get interrupted, this erases Flow, and it can take a while to get back into it.

Finding your flow is a great way to boost your happiness each day. How will you discover your flow today?

This now leads us to *The GLOW Ritual* **for Creative Flow**…

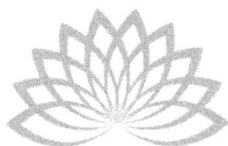

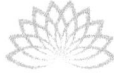

THE GLOW RITUAL
FOR CREATIVE FLOW

GRATITUDE & GET CREATIVE
Journaling Prompts

Today, write in your journal:

- What are your favourite things to do that make you feel in flow?
- How does this make you feel?
- How can you make more time to bring more flow into your life?
- Write down 5 things you are grateful for today?

LIVE HOLISTICALLY
Life Lessons

- Getting into a creative flow can help to build your confidence
- Finding your flow is a great happiness booster
- Immerse yourself with things that make you happy each day
- Discovering what you are good at gives you creative confidence in your abilities

ORGANISE YOUR LIFE
Get Organised

Today, finish a project that you have never got around to finishing. Maybe it is an art project, a DIY project or even finish or start writing that book you have always dreamed of. You cannot get organised when your mind is in multiple places at one time. So, get laser focused today on the one project you would like to complete.

TODAY'S MINI WELLNESS RITUAL

Today, do something that makes you feel in flow – where time stands still, and you feel relaxed and happy. It could be your favourite hobby, like yoga, art or making jewellery. Whatever it is, find your flow today.

I would love to see *The GLOW Ritual* you have decided to create for yourself today.

Don't forget to also tick each part of *The GLOW Ritual* off each day to support you in living your *Glowing Life Of Wellness*:

Gratitude & **G**et Creative
Live Holistically
Organise Your Life
Wellness Rituals

Share with me www.jaikooven.co.uk

DAY 10
A RITUAL FOR SELF-IMPROVEMENT

'Keep your heels, head, and standards high.'
Coco Chanel

FOCUS ON WHAT YOU CAN CHANGE

What could you change today that would make a difference to your life? Do you want to launch your own fashion range? If so, what courses can you take or what skills do you need to achieve that goal? Rather than feeling overwhelmed with the overall picture of the finished goal, e.g., to own your own fashion range, look at what you can do today to make a difference. When you focus on what you cannot change, you just feel frustrated and unmotivated. So, just focus on the little steps towards your goal and, in no time, you will achieve what you want in life.

As I write this chapter of this book, I understand the importance of the 'focus on what's within your power to change' message. You can get so busy focusing on the future or worrying about tomorrow that you forget to live for today.

CONTROL WHAT YOU CAN CONTROL

If you are worried about your job, worrying will get you nowhere. Instead focus on your work, make sure your CV is updated and maybe do a course in your spare time so that if you do lose your job, you have other options. If you are worried about getting ill, again worrying will cause your body to feel more stressed which won't help if you do get ill. So, just make sure you fill your body with healthy foods and vitamins and sanitise your hands if you are in public and keep yourself hygienic as possible. All of this is within your control. Also, if you ever did lose your job or get ill, then you would have known that you did everything you could beforehand to prevent these things from happening, and you would create a backup option in these circumstances of how you would tackle this scenario. Do not give your power away to anxiety and worry. Trust me when I say it does more harm than good. Worrying will equal more worrying.

THE SIX STAGES OF CHANGE

There are six stages of change, aka *The Transtheoretical Model*, which was developed by Prochaska and DiClemente in the late 1970s. The Transtheoretical Model (TTM) focuses on how individuals make decisions and their intention to change. The TTM suggests that individuals will go through the six stages below to get to the termination stage of their old habits. This process has always helped me when I have hit a block in my life and want to figure out a way forward and where I sit in the TTM. It also helps me when working with my clients and helping them to deal with their own blocks.

Here are the Six Stages of Change (aka The Transtheoretical Model):

1. **Not interested in changing a risky lifestyle (Precontemplation stage)**

At this stage, people will not be in the process to change and will not see that what they are doing in their daily lives is a problem. They do not intend to take action within the next six months to improve their situation. When at this stage, people will often not see the benefit to changing their behaviour and will place huge emphasis on the cons of them changing their behaviour at this time.

2. Thinking about Change (Contemplation Stage)

At this stage, people 'move on' and pass through the Precontemplation Stage. They begin to ponder whether the change would be of benefit to them and accept it as a potential option rather than eliminating it completely. People can recognize that their behaviour may be problematic, and they will start to weigh up the pros and cons with an equal emphasis on both. However, at this stage, they could equally revert back to the Precontemplation Stage.

3. Preparation (Determination Stage)

When people get to this stage it is because they feel they must change, and they must start making those changes right now. Over the next 30 days, people will start to take small steps forward towards their change to reach their goal. They believe that their behaviour change will lead to a happier and healthier life, so they are willing to take the step forward to do what it takes to change.

4. Making Changes (Action Stage)

At this stage, people have changed their behaviour within the last six months and intend to keep moving forward with their positive behaviour change. People may modify problems with their behaviour or acquire new healthy behaviours.

5. Breaking Down Old Behaviours (Maintenance Stage)

At this stage, people will have sustained their behaviour change for a more than six months and intend to carry on maintaining their new behaviour change. At this point, people will realise the importance of this stage in order not to relapse to previous stages.

6. New Beginnings (Termination Stage)

At this stage, there is no desire for the person to return to their old unhealthy behaviours and habits. They are sure that they will not relapse. This stage is often not considered in health promotion programs as people mainly stay in the maintenance stage as we are always learning and evolving.

So, where do you currently sit and what are you trying to change? How can you adapt to change for your self-improvement?

The things that I have been adapting and changing over the past few years have been many:

- Since my stepdad died in 2019, I learned a lot about myself and focused on my work to keep my mind occupied at such a traumatic time. On review, I worked too much and did not give myself a break because of feeling guilty, so this is where I will implement my new behaviour change – having a healthy work/life balance. I felt like I just wanted to make my stepdad proud, which in turn made me work harder.

- I realized the importance of slow living. As an author and International Holistic Expert, I always want to be learning and growing, but in doing so I burnt out my brain. I now understand the importance of slowing down. Life is not a race to get to the finish line whilst your life hangs in the balance. It is like being the Tortoise in the famous fable '*The Tortoise and the Hare*' - slow and steady wins the race. When you slow down, life has a different rhythm. You can hear the birds in the trees, and you live for the now. This is where I want to be. No more mind marathons for me!

- I discovered how to find the joy in the little things. Years ago, I was quite materialistic. I would find the greatest joy when I acquired the latest designer handbag or next clothing item, yet inside I would feel empty. I did not appreciate the little things in life and realise that true happiness does not lie in buying a handbag. Now, I appreciate every little thing I have; my health, my home, my family and my career. I have made it my mission over the years to appreciate all the little joys in life, rather than trying to find joy in things that do not matter. I work my hardest every day to find joy in the simplest of things and that makes me so happy.

- I believe that I can achieve and be anything I want to be in life. This belief in myself is what inspires me to always do better and constantly grow as a person. I will always be maintaining this healthy habit as it helps me to achieve my goals in life and not feel stuck. I know I can achieve all I set out to do with a plan and I feel truly inspired to follow my dreams in life. One of my dreams was to write this book and it is the most amazing thing to achieve this lifelong dream.

- I recently got a little puppy - an eight-week-old Maltese Shih Tzu (Malshi in short). I realized how beneficial it is to have her in my life and in my family. She brings me so much joy and is full of affection. She helps me to stay grounded and grateful that the simplest things in life can make you happy. I love her warmth and unconditional love that she gives to me and the overall sense of happiness and wellbeing that I feel when I am around her.

You do not appreciate your health until it is gone. You do not appreciate your health until you can no longer reverse the damage that is done. Why should it take a big scare like cancer to change the way you eat, think and behave? I really appreciate my health and wellbeing every day and it is always at the very top of my to do list. I do not feel guilty about putting my self-care first as I realise how precious my life really is.

When you focus on improving your situation and appreciating everything you have rather than moaning about things, your life completely changes. You start to look for every little thing to be thankful for and, rather than live in lack, you live a life of abundance every single day

This now leads us to *The GLOW Ritual* for Self-Improvement…

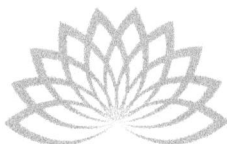

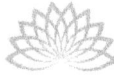

THE GLOW RITUAL
FOR SELF-IMPROVEMENT

GRATITUDE & GET CREATIVE
Journaling Prompts

Today, write in your journal:

- List 5 areas in your life that you would like to improve
- Pick one to focus on and write down why this matters to you
- What date would you like to achieve this by and why?
- Write down 5 things you are grateful for today

LIVE HOLISTICALLY
Life Lessons

- Focusing on what you can change gives you the confidence to make a change
- When you focus on what you don't have, or focus on lack, then it acts as a block for your abundance
- Life is not a race to the finishing line - you are always improving and growing

ORGANISE YOUR LIFE
Get Organised

Today, what in your life would you like to improve? Would you like to get fitter or healthier? Would you like to read more books? Whatever it is, dedicate yourself to doing something for your self-improvement today. If you are feeling more motivated, do it for 30 days.

WELLNESS RITUALS
Time For Self-Care

Today, hydrate with warm water and lemon. Water is so important for the healthy functioning of our nervous system and to support our body to function properly. A classic Ayurvedic remedy of warm water and lemon will help to boost your immune system with a burst of Vitamin C and will help to give your mood and metabolism a boost too.

I would love to see *The GLOW Ritual* you have decided to create for yourself today.

Don't forget to also tick each part of *The GLOW Ritual* off each day to support you in living your *Glowing Life Of Wellness*:

Gratitude & Get Creative
Live Holistically
Organise Your Life
Wellness Rituals

Share with me www.jaikooven.co.uk

THE SACRAL CHAKRA RITUALS

In this chapter, we covered:

- *The GLOW Ritual* of Healing Your Inner Child
- *The GLOW Ritual* of New Beginnings
- *The GLOW Ritual* of Empowerment
- *The GLOW Ritual* of Creative Flow
- *The GLOW Ritual* of Self-Improvement

This chapter describes the building blocks to your creative talents. We covered how to heal your inner child wounds, so you can boost your creative confidence and achieve your goals in life.

THE SACRAL CHAKRA

In this section, we covered all information about the Sacral Chakra. The Sacral Chakra supports you in expressing yourself freely through your creativity. This allows you to feel inspired and encourages you to gain creative confidence so you can create positive changes in your life, on all levels.

When you are stuck and out of balance with your Sacral Chakra, you can feel creatively blocked or find it hard to relax into the flow of life.

The Sacral Chakra is about bringing more creative fun into your life and being passionate about the things you do.

SACRAL CHAKRA CRYSTALS:

Carnelian
Carnelian is the overall crystal balancer for this Chakra as it is a great crystal for motivation and creativity. It encourages us to embrace vitality in our lives by living in the present moment.

Sunstone
Sunstone is great for boosting your self-confidence and boosting your Sacral and Solar Plexus Chakras and supporting you with strength and enthusiasm in your new goals.

Citrine
Citrine helps to give you joyful energy and makes you feel more positive. It is also a great crystal for attracting abundance.

ESSENTIAL OILS FOR THE SACRAL CHAKRA:

Use an essential oil diffuser to surround yourself with a choice of one of these scents or create your own uplifting mixture.

PLEASE SEEK MEDICAL OR PROFESSIONAL ADVICE IF YOU ARE PREGNANT OR HAVE A MEDICAL CONDITION.

Sweet Orange Oil

Sweet orange oil is great for making you feel uplifted and happy. It is refreshing and encourages fun, joy and creativity as it is also known as the 'Smiley Oil'.

Jasmine

Jasmine is a great essential oil for confidence and optimism. It brings a sense of euphoria to your mind and helps you feel more confident when tackling larger projects.

Frankincense

Frankincense is the essential oil for calming and soothing the mind, body *and* spirit. It is a nurturing oil that allows us to gain creative clarity.

REFLECTION

When you look at your current life now, how can you bring more creativity into your days? What inner child healing would you like to continue to work on so you can gain more confidence in those areas as an adult?

POSITIVE CHANGE

With the knowledge you have gained, what three creative goals would you like to work on over the next three months?

Well done on completing your second Chakra Chapter on the Sacral Chakra.

What did you enjoy the most about this chapter? Let me know at www.jaikooven.co.uk and don't forget to share your daily mini rituals too.

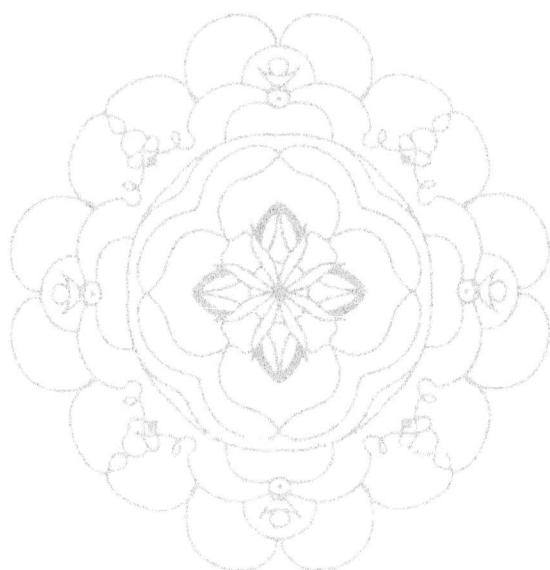

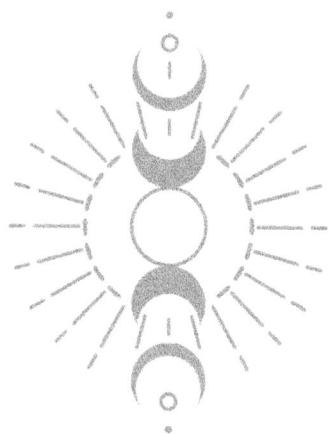

Glow with Joy

❀

CHAPTER

Three

SOLAR PLEXUS CHAKRA

THE SOLAR PLEXUS CHAKRA

The Solar Plexus is also referred to as *Manipura* (meaning 'shining gem', 'seat of gems' or 'city of jewels'). It is the Chakra for joy, abundance and personal strength. When your Solar Plexus is aligned, it helps you to build your self-esteem, set healthy boundaries and have the willpower to succeed. A balanced Solar Plexus also allows you to adapt to change in your life.

The Solar Plexus is the Chakra for you to embrace your personal power. It gives you a sense of self-worth and is the foundation of your inner guidance. You know in your gut that you are on the right path, and you follow your intuition.

WHERE IS THE SOLAR PLEXUS LOCATED?

The Solar Plexus is located in the centre of your abdomen.

WHAT COLOUR IS THE SOLAR PLEXUS?

Yellow

HOW WILL I FEEL IF THIS CHAKRA IS BALANCED?

- You will be able to express your core values

- You will be able to manage your emotions, thoughts and instincts

- You will have determination to succeed

- You will have strong boundaries

- You will be dedicated to your life path

- You have trust within yourself and your inner guidance

- You feel inspired by others, not jealous

- You don't need external validation

HOW MIGHT I FEEL IF I AM OUT OF BALANCE?

- You may feel in 'victim mode' and powerless

- You may misuse your power to manipulate others

- You may find it hard to take action to pursue your goals

- You may have low esteem

- You may suffer from stomach discomfort and anxiety

SELF-LOVE WAYS TO GET BACK IN BALANCE

- Wear yellow or eat yellow foods which are healthy e.g., bananas, starfruit, sweetcorn or melon

- Do a Solar Plexus Chakra Yoga Class or meditation through YouTube or through my membership programme

- Step out of your comfort zone

- Have confidence in yourself and your decision-making process

- Spend time in the sunshine.

DAY 11
A RITUAL FOR SELF-DISCLIPINE

'Live as if you were to die tomorrow.
Learn as if you were to live forever.'
Mahatma Gandhi

BEING DETERMINED TO SUCCEED

In the *Yoga Sutras of Patañjali*, an ancient text that is the foundation of yoga philosophy, two of the 'Eight Limbs of Yoga' are the *Yamas* and *Niyamas*. These are guidelines for how to live your life. One of the *Niyamas* is *Tapas*, or self-discipline. This is our focused effort to become someone of determined strength and strong character. To make a short-term sacrifice for a long-term gain. My book ***The GLOW Ritual*** is a prime example of *Tapas*.

I have worked endlessly on this book for around 18 months, for hours on end, with determination that I will have a published book by the end of this process. It is with self-discipline and consistency that you will succeed in anything in your life, and that is what has helped me to stay motivated during this time.

At times it has been extremely hard, like running a marathon when you feel you have nothing left to give. At other times, like yoga, it flows beautifully. This is just life, and it is my strong self-discipline at this time that has kept me going because I really wanted this book to support and inspire people all around the world.

With all things in life, from losing weight to writing a book, if you really want them, take a little effort day by day to improve a little at a time.

For example, many yo-yo dieters put the weight back on

quickly. A diet is not a quick fix - it is a lifestyle change. If you can create a healthy lifestyle, then your body will maintain a healthy weight. If you go on a salad diet for a month and lose a lot of weight, then binge on chocolate the next month, this is you self-sabotaging yourself.

Therefore, I believe in creating daily rituals in your life that keep you empowered and grounded. Empowerment will help you keep focused on your goals and keep you feeling confident about achieving what you want in life. By staying grounded, you can also stay connected with your wellbeing. I liken this to the *Yin and Yang* energies that I discuss further on in this book. The action of doing and just being. Finding the perfect balance of self-care and self-discipline to get you where you want in life.

No matter what you want in life, it starts with a plan. Ask yourself: What do you want? When do you want it? How will you get it? Then work out your daily actionable plan from there and do not give up. Be consistent with your efforts and, if you fall off track, quickly get back on. Acknowledge your time for rest as well as your time to keep moving and I promise you, one day things will finally click and you will look back and see how much you have achieved and how far you have come.

It is easy to become overwhelmed with anything when you get started. You compare your day one to somebody else's 20 years of experience and you wonder, *How the hell will I ever get there*? But EVERYONE starts at day one at some point on their journey. Why not start yours today?

This now leads us to **The GLOW Ritual for Self-Discipline**...

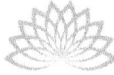

THE GLOW RITUAL
FOR SELF-DISCLIPLINE

GRATITUDE & GET CREATIVE
Journaling Prompts

Today, write in your journal:

- What areas in your life could you be more self-disciplined?
- Write down your wellness ritual today and plan how you will do it daily to get your desired result
- With your plan, now work out when you want to achieve that goal, so you can create daily rituals to make it happen.
- Write down 5 things you are grateful for today

LIVE HOLISTICALLY
Life Lessons

- Learn to do what it takes to get the results you want in your life
- Have the determination to succeed and never give up on your dreams
- When you are focused with your goals in life, you can achieve anything you want

ORGANISE YOUR LIFE
Get Organised

Today, how can you improve your self-discipline to get what you want. Do you want to lose weight? Run a marathon? Start your first day of self-discipline today to get you what you want. Plan your strategy to support you in your self-discipline today.

WELLNESS RITUALS
Time For Self-Care

Today, as you are working on your focus and self-discipline, give art therapy a try. Art therapy is a great form of self-care and has been proven to help people clarify their emotions, reduce anxiety and improve self-awareness. It is a great way to express your creative expression too. A few examples of art therapy are adult colouring, painting a DIY project or drawing. What will you create?

I would love to see *The GLOW Ritual* you have decided to create for yourself today.

Don't forget to also tick each part of *The GLOW Ritual* off each day to support you in living your *Glowing Life Of Wellness*:

Gratitude & **G**et Creative
Live Holistically
Organise Your Life
Wellness Rituals

Share with me www.jaikooven.co.uk

DAY 12
A RITUAL FOR MOTIVATION

'The only impossible journey is the one you never begin.'
Tony Robbins

MOVING FORWARDS

Between the year 2020 to 2021, I moved house, travelled to six countries, went through three national lockdowns because of Covid-19, launched my own stationery range, worked with dozens of clients, gained another eight qualifications and started writing for a national magazine. On top of that, I also launched The Mind Spa Membership – an online wellness membership for the busy modern woman that includes daily yoga, meditation, self-care advice, sound healing and much more. I collaborated with the most amazing people and welcomed some inspiring spiritual teachers into my life. I read over 52 books that year, as well as being a mum. I also achieved an amazing goal of launching my debut and best-selling oracle card deck that I had been dreaming of doing for years. Lastly, I wrote this book as well as started planning two others.

ANYTHING IS POSSIBLE

None of this happened by magic. It involved disciplined daily action, lots of motivation and sacrifice. I would often ask myself whether the actions I was taking would take me to where I wanted to be. What did the person I wanted to be look like and what did she do on a daily basis? I literally became the person that I wanted to become in mind, body and spirit. I took action everyday and I looked after my wellbeing. I absorbed information like a sponge and applied it to my own daily life and business. I decided that I wanted to be a magnet for success and that I would draw success to me in any way I could. I would manifest everything I wanted in life, just by taking action each day.

'The Ritual of Motivation' involves just that - being motivated to take action every day so you can know you are achieving what you want in your life. Whether that is achieving an empty washing basket or closing a big business deal, by taking action and not being overwhelmed with the steps to success, you can get there. Little and often. It is a bit like exercise really; some people get a burst of inspiration and decide they want to run 5k. They do it, then realise that it's over and don't do it again. By being motivated to take daily action, you are making progress every day. It is not the fastest to the finish line but rather it is the slow steps that lead to the longest wins in life which can help you make your dreams come true.

MAKING THE IMPOSSIBLE POSSIBLE

When I was younger and as I was growing up, I would often come up with a 'crazy' idea about a business venture or career that I wanted to do. My mum would often say "Mum knows best", and that my idea was too risky, so I needed to be careful or just not try in case I failed or there was too much competition out there.

This would often leave me feeling frustrated, unsupported and I felt like my ideas were creatively suppressed. However, that never stopped me from pursuing my ideas, no matter how 'crazy' they were. Now that I am a Mum, I realise that the reason she said those things was to try to protect me from failure and disappointment, and it was her way of keeping me safe.

However, as a Cancerian, I am highly intuitive, and I knew from a young age that I would not take a traditional route in my life. My mum did not realise that to me, you have failed in life if you do not try in the first place. If you are truly happy with a regular 9-5 job, then if that works for you, then great! But I would rather be filling up my own soul's cup everyday doing a job that fulfils me in every way and excites me. I love the fact that when I start work each morning, I am making a difference in people's lives.

I live with purpose every day because the things that I create can inspire people's lives and make a difference. I work with beautiful women and empower them to feel holistically whole, as well as creatively confident to do something truly amazing in this world. I follow my soul's calling every day and nothing could be more rewarding than that.

My greatest life lesson that I would like to teach you today is to never play small. Do not listen to the naysayers that say you can't. I have spent years and will spend the rest of my living days proving to everyone that I can and so can you!

You may weave through uncertain paths and try lots of different jobs because you are trying to find where your talents lie. That is perfectly fine, you are only trying to find your way. I promise you that when you find your soul's true calling, you will know and everyday will be in alignment with you being authentically yourself and being recognized for your talent and energy that you put into your role.

You will wake up every day feeling connected to the person you want to be and stand proud of who you are. Your perfect job or life is not about watching '*A Day in My Life*' videos on YouTube which are very often filtered and unrealistic for people that have family and other commitments. It is waking up every day knowing that if you died tomorrow, you stood true to who you are and what you wanted to do in this world. No money or promotion in a job will ever give you the empowered and contented feeling you get when you know that, no matter what, you have chosen the right path for you.

My amazing late stepdad always made the impossible possible. There was no doubt in his mind that you could do or be anything you wanted in life. So, I will always carry his legacy forwards to make you feel that anything is possible for you too and to never ever give up. I would rather die trying than fail living a life I do not want to live. Sadly, my late stepdad died at age 56. He finally got to retirement after working a very stressful corporate job for many years and he enjoyed his retirement for one year before he died. We often put all our hopes and dreams into when we retire rather than doing everything we ever dreamed of doing now. What if there was no tomorrow? How would you make your dreams come true today?

Everything is possible if you try and truly believe you can. You just have to find a way to make it happen and stay motivated on your journey towards your success.

This now leads us to today's **The GLOW Ritual for Motivation**…

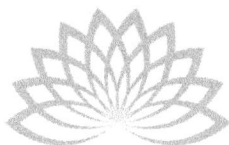

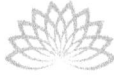

THE GLOW RITUAL
FOR MOTIVATION

GRATITUDE & GET CREATIVE
Journaling Prompts

Today, write in your journal:

- What will you do today to make the impossible possible?
- What would make you feel like you are living your life in alignment with your soul's true calling?
- Write down 5 things you are grateful for today

LIVE HOLISTICALLY
Life Lessons

- Learning to always move forwards in a positive way
- Anything is possible when you believe you can
- Believe in yourself and never play small
- Live a life with purpose and be proud of who you are

ORGANISE YOUR LIFE
Get Organised

Today, grab a bin bag and go around your house doing a 15-minute declutter challenge. You will be amazed at how much lighter and revitalized you feel and will have a tidier and clean home too because of it. You will be making a difference to charities too by donating your unwanted belongings.

WELLNESS RITUALS
Time For Self-Care

Today, live your life as if your dreams have already come true. Act out your whole day as if you have got your dream job or house or lost the weight you wanted to lose. This is a great confidence booster and is very inspiring for times when you are feeling unmotivated or lost in your purpose.

I would love to see *The GLOW Ritual* you have decided to create for yourself today.

Don't forget to also tick each part of *The GLOW Ritual* off each day to support you in living your *Glowing Life Of Wellness*:

Gratitude & **G**et Creative
Live Holistically
Organise Your Life
Wellness Rituals

Share with me www.jaikooven.co.uk

DAY 13
A RITUAL FOR HAPPINESS HABITS

'Happiness is the best makeup.'
Drew Barrymore

WHAT IS HAPPINESS?

At our core, we just want to be happy and live a fulfilling life. It is not about finding your happiness in the next luxury car or designer handbag purchase; it is about finding the happiness within yourself.

It sounds simple, but people spend their lives in pursuit of happiness, and they never find it.

When you go in search of happiness, it will elude you. It is not something that can be found, it is something that you create for yourself. You can decide to be happier and this can make you feel happier. With a positive mindset you can learn to be happier and not place your happiness on a person or materialistic item to provide that happiness for you. When you seek happiness anywhere else but within, it will always be short-lived and you can end up disappointed. True happiness that you find within yourself, you can have in abundance.

I studied a course in Happiness when I had PTSD, and I remember it saying that the happiest people are optimistic and have a positive mindset and outlook on life. They see the silver lining in everything, and they focus on what they have, rather than what they lack. Any problem is no problem to them as they will always see the good that came out of that situation.

Happy people cultivate a healthy habit of gratitude. They are thankful for their lives and everything they have in it. Their lives may not be perfect, but they are grateful for what they are blessed with each day. They do not take things for granted and are consistently grateful for everything they have in their lives.

Letting go of bad feelings and negative energy is another way that you can manage your happiness levels.

When we live in the present, rather than the past or future, our happiness can also be always present. Your mind is not stuck in the past or the future as it is purely finding happiness in the now, so you can enjoy every moment as it is.

When you live in line with your values and are authentically yourself, you will find that you are happier. When you try to please others, or compare yourself to others on social media, this can cause you a huge amount of anxiety and feelings of inadequacy. Constantly comparing yourself with others can lead you to constantly feeling like you are in a never-ending comparison cycle.

STOP COMPARING YOURSELF

I found my true happiness and confidence within myself when I stopped comparing myself to others. There will always be someone who may be better than you in some way and there will always be someone that is not as good as you in other ways. That does not mean that you are any less or more deserving of finding your happiness in your own talents. When you believe in yourself, you become your own best friend and you know 100% those great rewards will come to you if you put the effort in.

A great way to boost your happiness in this way is to focus on your wins and how far you have come rather than how far you need to go and celebrate every achievement, no matter how big or small. This way, you are able to acknowledge your self-worth, rather than belittling your achievements.

We all make mistakes and that is how we learn and grow as people. So, having self-acceptance of a situation will help you find your happiness again. If something matters to you, do not get down if you fail the first time. Just keep on trying and you will get there in the end.

Surround yourself with other happy people as this will give you good and positive energy and lift your mood. Happiness is a feel-good vibe and is contagious, so when you are with happy people, it makes you feel happy also. We mirror the people around us.

HAPPINESS AND SOCIAL MEDIA

Sadly, our social media is packed with people showing their 'perfect' and often fake lives. I have come to realise, over the years of studying various holistic therapies and psychology, that the happiest people are the people that feel they have nothing to prove. They do not announce their 'perfect relationship' on social media because instead they are enjoying their 'perfect relationship'. They are not posting to seek approval or acknowledgement for the things that they buy or how they look, or posting pictures of themselves in their underwear for all to see. Finding true happiness is about connection and not about posting to strangers who do not matter. Therefore, often many people on social media are suffering from anxiety, depression and self-esteem issues, because they are trying to prove their worth to people that do not matter.

GETTING YOUR DAILY DOSE OF VITAMIN J

The best way of finding happiness is to give back to others as it makes you feel like you are making a difference. Getting your daily dose of Vitamin J (Joy) is a great way to boost your happiness levels.

Creativity is a great skill to promote joy, and this is why I included it in your daily **GLOW Ritual – Gratitude & Get Creative**. We are all creative in some way and creativity is a great outlet for self-expression. The art of creating something beautiful, whether it is art or redecorating your home, is a great way of finding happiness and fulfilment.

Meditation and mindfulness practices are fantastic for increasing your joy levels. Whether it is through seated meditation or a simple mindfulness practice, you will get the same results. You learn how to tune into what is going on in your mind and you learn how to find peace by detaching yourself from your ego and emotions.

Exercising is one of the best ways to boost your happiness. That is why happy people exercise regularly. When you exercise, your body releases endorphins which trigger positive emotions which make you feel happy. You also feel good for achieving something positive and because you are taking care of your body. It also helps alleviate stress in your body and your mind. If you are feeling down, try taking a walk or do a yoga session and you will notice that your mood will improve dramatically.

It is important to realise that your everyday happiness is already yours to claim, and it all starts with a smile and a grateful heart each day.

This now leads us to today's *The GLOW Ritual* **for Happiness Habits**…

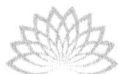

THE GLOW RITUAL
FOR HAPPINESS HABITS

GRATITUDE & GET CREATIVE
Journaling Prompts

Today, write in your journal:

- List 5 things that make you happy.
- What makes you feel truly happy?
- Write down 5 things you are grateful for today

LIVE HOLISTICALLY
Life Lessons

- Happiness cannot be bought
- You have to find happiness within yourself and not seek it externally
- Stop comparing yourself to others and find happiness from where you are right now

ORGANISE YOUR LIFE
Get Organised

From the 5 things that make you happy that you wrote down in your journal, how can you get organised so you can apply those things to each day?

WELLNESS RITUALS
Time For Self-Care

Today, do something that will make you really happy.
Whether it is riding your bike, reading a book or watching
an inspiring film. What can you do today to bring you
joy?

I would love to see *The GLOW Ritual* you have decided
to create for yourself today.

Don't forget to also tick each part of *The GLOW Ritual*
off each day to support you in living your *Glowing Life
Of Wellness*:

Gratitude & **G**et Creative
Live Holistically
Organise Your Life
Wellness Rituals

Share with me www.jaikooven.co.uk

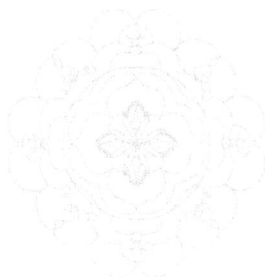

DAY 14
A RITUAL FOR POSITIVITY

'If you light a lamp for somebody,
it will also brighten your path.'
Buddha

BE A GOAL GETTER

I sometime hear people ask, "Why should anyone have goals?" Well, there are quite a few reasons, but to put it in a nutshell, goal setting really does help you to plan, and when you have a plan, you can do something about it. That is what helps make your dreams become your reality.

By putting a plan into action, you can make it happen. It is all in the doing! The process of setting goals helps you choose where you want to go in life. By knowing precisely what you want to achieve, you know where you must concentrate your efforts. You'll also quickly spot the distractions that would otherwise lure you from your course.

When I introduced daily, weekly and monthly goals into my life, my whole life changed and yours can too.

Here are some steps to help you get started in achieving your goals:

TEN STEPS TO ACHIEVING YOUR GOALS

1. What exactly do you want? Define your goal.

Is your goal clearly defined with a specific plan of action? Is it important to you personally? Is it within your power to make happen? Is it something you have a reasonable chance of achieving?

Are you clear about what is important for you in your life? Do you make your choices based on this?

You can only achieve your goals if you are totally clear on exactly what it is you want.

2. How strong is your desire? Determine the strength of your desire. Do your goals inspire and energize you?

On a scale of 1 -10, with 1 being very weak and 10 being 'I'd do anything to achieve this goal,' how strong is your desire?

Is your goal something YOU really want or is it something you think, or you've been told you should want?

The greater your desire, the stronger your inner drive to action towards that goal.

3. Have you written down your goals? If not, write them down.

Have you put your goal on paper and made it official? Did you know that only 3 % of people write down their goals, but of those 3%, 80% of them actually achieve their goals? Are you one of the 80%?

Writing down your goal is your declaration that You Want It! Be specific. Place it where you will see it several times a day

4. Can you see and feel yourself having what you want? Define all the ways you will benefit from reaching your goal.

Can you visualize yourself having arrived at your goal?

Where are you? How is your life different? What are you doing? How do you feel? Be specific.

The more benefits you can envision, the more energized and inspired you will feel and the greater the pull that goal will have on you. See and feel yourself already there. Use the power of that vision to fuel your actions.

5. Where are you now? Determine your starting point.

What is your starting point? Do you know where you are now, in order to plot the most advantageous and direct course to your destination? With a clear starting point, you can head in the right direction. Making a plan is much like mapping your route for a road trip - if you don't know where you are, you can't know how to get to where you are going.

6. What is your time frame? Set timelines and deadlines.

Have you committed to timelines and deadlines? Are you MAKING the time to MAKE the goal? Have you scheduled time to work on your goal and put that time into your diary? Have you prioritized and eliminated things that are of less, or no, value? By doing this, you commit to clearing the way to taking action towards your goal.

7. What obstacles might you face and how will you deal with them? Consider possible blocks/obstacles and ways of dealing with them.

What possible obstacles will you face? Have you prepared contingency plans to deal with those obstacles? How can you deal with them the most effectively? If you are prepared, then you will know how to overcome this obstacles when they stand in your way.

8. What are your strengths and resources? Identify resources.

What strengths and resources do you have that will help you move forward? Who are the people or organizations that will support you? Who is on your success team? How can you improve the skills you'll need and build on the strengths you already have? Have you succeeded or failed at tasks that were similar to this before? What resources did you use that were helpful before? What can you do to maximize your chances of success this time? What can you do differently? What can you do to motivate yourself to reach your goal? Be your own best resource.

9. What is your plan and what are the steps? Make a plan.

> *'A dream is just a dream. A goal is a dream with a plan and a deadline.'*
>
> *Harvey MacKay*

Have you broken your goal down into small manageable steps that can be done daily? Have you identified and time-lined each task that needs to be done? Have you discerned your starting point? What do you need to do first? What structures do you have in place to keep track of your progress? Accomplishing a goal requires taking the steps. These steps, in turn, become habits. What daily habits do you need to create? Big successes start with little ones.

10. Are you committed? Make a commitment and believe in yourself.

Are you committed or are you just trying? How many people do you know who have tried to do something and failed?

Say the following sentence to yourself: "I'm going to try to _____ "

Now say, "I'm committed to _____ "

Which feels more solid and more likely to happen? To achieve any goal, you need to COMMIT yourself to achieving it. Have you really committed to doing every single thing that's necessary to achieve that goal? Are you committed to putting in ALL the necessary time, energy and money?

Look over your plan and the steps to achieve your goal. Do you believe that you can do it? Do you have any doubts? Are your expectations realistic?

Deal with your fears and expectations of yourself. Remind yourself that you can and will do this.

Bonus Step: Celebrate

How will you acknowledge the work that you have done and celebrate the completion of each of the steps along the way? How can you use that energy of success to keep you moving forward? Don't wait until the end to celebrate.

Celebrating each small victory acknowledges your successes and keeps you motivated and focused. As well as having goals, you have to understand 'The Power of Positivity'.

THE POWER OF POSITIVITY

I am going to ask you something very weird right now. First of all, I want you to listen to your thoughts. Now tell me, what thoughts fill your head? Would you label them as positive, or negative?

Now let's say you are walking down the street with these thoughts. Do you think anyone who met you would be able to tell you what's on your mind?

The answer to number one is up to you, but the answer to number two can be pretty generic. Although people will not be able to tell you exactly what you think, they will usually more or less have an idea of how you are feeling as they can pick up on your energy.

Thoughts are very powerful. They affect your general attitude. The attitude you carry reflects on your appearance too, unless of course, you are a great actor.

And it doesn't end there. Your attitude can also affect people around you. The type of attitude you carry depends on you. It can be either positive or negative.

Positive thoughts can make you feel invigorated. Plus, the people around the person carrying positive thoughts are usually energized by this type of attitude too.

Negative thoughts, on the other hand, have a sapping effect on other people. Aside from making you look gloomy and sad, negative thoughts can turn a festive gathering into a funeral wake.

A positive attitude attracts people, while a negative attitude repels them. People tend to shy away from those who carry a negative attitude.

We can also define attitude as the way of looking at the world. If you choose to focus on the negative things in the world, you have a negative attitude brewing up. However, if you choose to focus on the positive things, you are more likely to carry a positive attitude.

You have much to gain from a very positive attitude. For

one, studies have shown that a positive attitude promotes better health. Those with this kind of attitude also have more friends. Projecting a positive attitude also helps people handle stress and problems better than those who have a negative attitude.

A positive attitude begins with a healthy self-image. If you love the way you are and are satisfied, confident, and self-assured, you also make others around you feel the same way.

On the other hand, a negative attitude had an opposite effect. So, carrying a negative attitude has a twofold drawback; you feel bad about yourself, and you make others feel the same way.

If you want to have a positive attitude, you need to feature healthy thoughts. This is often harder to do nowadays since, all around us, the media feeds us nothing but negative thoughts. A study shows that for every 14 things a parent says to his or her child, only one is positive. This is truly a saddening thought.

Although it is impossible to keep ourselves from the negative things around us, you can still carry a positive attitude by focusing on the good things and the positive things in life.

This positive attitude you now carry can be of benefit to other people. Sometimes, when others feel down, the thing people mostly do is try to give them advice. But sometimes, all they need is somebody to sit by them and listen to them. If you have a positive attitude, you may be able to cheer them up without even having to say anything.

If a positive attitude is lovely, why do people choose to adopt a negative attitude instead? Those who carry a negative attitude may be actually sending a signal for attention. Before you get me wrong, feeling sad, angry, or gloomy is not wrong in itself. However, dwelling on these thoughts for too long is not healthy either. There is a time to mourn.

As always, if you are beset by troubles, even in your darkest hour, focus on the good things in life and you will always have hope. Problems become something you can overcome rather than a constant battle

You do not have anything to lose by adopting a healthy, positive attitude. Studies show that such an attitude actually reverses ageing, makes you healthier, helps you develop a better stress coping mechanism, and has a very positive effect on all the people you meet every day. So, what's not to like about a positive attitude? Adopt one today.

Negativity shows all around, starting from the inside and making its way to your physical appearance. So, bring more sunshine into your days with a more positive attitude. See what amazing things you attract into your life and how great it makes you feel from the inside out.

This now leads us to today's *The GLOW Ritual* **for Positivity**…

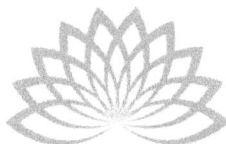

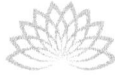

THE GLOW RITUAL
FOR POSITIVITY

GRATITUDE & GET CREATIVE
Journaling Prompts

Today, write in your journal:

* List 6 goals you would like to achieve in the next months
* Individually work out how you will achieve them
* Write down a reward if you achieve all 6
* Write down 5 things you are grateful for today

LIVE HOLISTICALLY
Life Lessons

* Even in your darkest moments, focus on the light. A positive mindset has power in your life
* Learn to define what is your plan and what are your steps to achieving your goals

ORGANISE YOUR LIFE
Get Organised

Today, you are going to get organised with your thoughts. What negative thoughts are getting stuck in your mind? Write them out in your journal and then write out the positive version of each of your negative thoughts. This is a great way to shift your mindset and focus on the positive things in your life.

WELLNESS RITUALS
Time For Self-Care

Now you have decluttered your mind, how can you bring more positivity into your day? Your aim today is to be as positive as possible. Surround yourself with positivity and do not speak in a negative way. Explore how this feels for you.

I would love to see *The GLOW Ritual* you have decided to create for yourself today.

Don't forget to also tick each part of *The GLOW Ritual* off each day to support you in living your *Glowing Life Of Wellness*:

Gratitude & Get Creative
Live Holistically
Organise Your Life
Wellness Rituals

Share with me www.jaikooven.co.uk

THE SOLAR PLEXUS CHAKRA

CHAPTER SUMMARY

In this chapter, we covered:

- *The GLOW Ritual* for Self-Discipline
- *The GLOW Ritual* for Motivation
- *The GLOW Ritual* for Happiness Habits
- *The GLOW Ritual* for Positivity

This chapter covered your personal strength and encouraged you to bring positive changes into your life. The Solar Plexus supports you in building self-esteem, setting personal boundaries and supporting you with your willpower. It supports you in bringing positive changes into your life.

REFLECTION

When you look at your current life, what could you change to be more disciplined with your goals? What improvements could you make to improve your happiness levels?

POSITIVE CHANGE

Write down in a journal three things that you have learnt from this chapter that you will now incorporate into your daily life going forwards.

CRYSTALS FOR SOLAR PLEXUS CHAKRA

Amazonite

Amazonite is one of my favourite crystals. Not only is it beautiful to look at, but it allows you to enjoy happier relationships and tune into our intuition. It also allows us to make healthier decisions that can lead to our overall happiness.

Citrine

Citrine helps to give you joyful energy and makes you feel more positive. It is also a great crystal for attracting abundance.

Amethyst

Amethyst is a beautiful and calming crystal. It helps to keep us centred whilst also uplifting us.

ESSENTIAL OILS FOR THE SOLAR PLEXUS CHAKRA

Use an essential oil diffuser to surround yourself with a choice of one of these scents or create your own uplifting mixture.

PLEASE SEEK MEDICAL OR PROFESSIONAL ADVICE IF YOU ARE PREGNANT OR HAVE A MEDICAL CONDITION.

Lavender

Lavender essential oil is very popular for relaxation. It helps with anxiety and stress. It also has an uplifting effect that boosts your overall happiness levels.

Bergamot

Bergamot essential oil is great for supporting you in alleviating work-related stress by reducing feelings of anxiety and making you feel more relaxed and happier.

Jasmine

Jasmine is one of my favourite essential oils and is really popular in perfumes. Jasmine promotes a wonderful feeling of wellbeing and happiness. It also makes you feel more romantic and energetic.

Well done on completing your third chapter on the Solar Plexus Chakra.

What did you enjoy the most about this chapter? Let me know at www.jaikooven.co.uk and don't forget to share your daily mini rituals too.

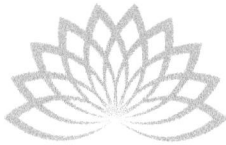

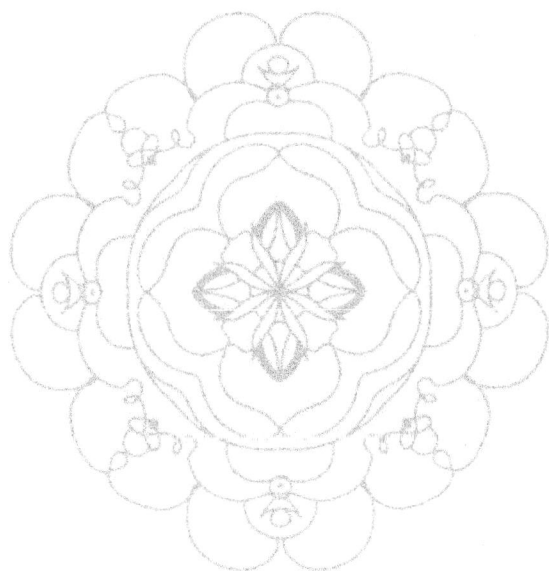

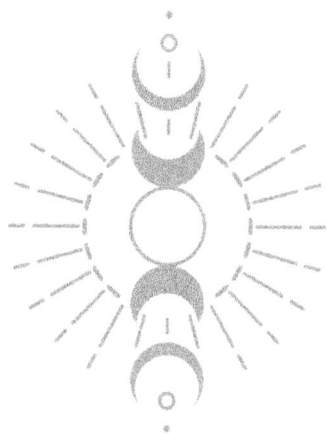

Glow with Self-Love

CHAPTER

Four

PINK HEART CHAKRA

THE PINK HEART CHAKRA

In *The GLOW Ritual*, I have decided to incorporate two Heart Chakras, as I thought it was important to balance the masculine and feminine aspects of this Chakra. The Heart Chakra is also referred to as *Anahata* which in Sanskrit means 'unhurt', 'unbeaten' and 'unstruck'.

The Heart Chakra is associated with serenity, calmness and balance in your life. It is also associated with unconditional love.

The Pink Heart Chakra supports the divine feminine energy which supports healing past hurts, relationships and grief.

WHERE IS THE PINK HEART CHAKRA LOCATED?

The Pink Heart Chakra is located in the centre of the chest, in the region of the heart.

WHAT COLOUR IS THE PINK HEART CHAKRA?

Pink.

HOW WILL I FEEL IF THIS CHAKRA IS BALANCED?

- You will radiate love

- You will feel calm and at peace

- You will make time for your own self-love and care

- You will have self-care and beauty regimes to help you feel beautifully balanced

HOW MIGHT I FEEL IF I AM OUT OF BALANCE?

- You cannot heal your past wounds and life experiences

- You may feel disharmony in your life through grief or sadness

- You may find it hard to give or receive love

SELF-LOVE WAYS TO GET BACK IN BALANCE

- Wear pink

- Have a self-care day and visit a spa

- Go on a romantic date

- Buy a Rose Quartz crystal from my crystal shop

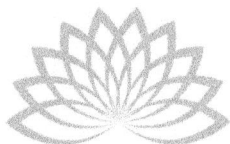

DAY 15
A RITUAL FOR SELF-LOVE

'Love is the great miracle cure. Loving ourselves works miracles in our lives.'
Louise Hay

SHOWING YOURSELF SOME SELF-CARE

Self-love is also defined as 'love of self' and it means taking care of your own wellbeing and happiness.

Showing yourself some self-love through self-care is such a rewarding thing for your wellbeing. We often don't realise the importance of self-care until it is too late, and we have burnt ourselves out.

When was the last time someone asked you if you were 'looking after yourself'? Can you honestly say that you are?

Too often, we place too much pressure on ourselves, or we expect too much of ourselves. We are constantly working hard toward our goals, and we beat ourselves up if we are anything other than perfect in that pursuit.

Is it any surprise we are often over-tired, malnourished, and depressed?

Self-care comes in all forms and can include:

- Time for reading

- Time with friends

- A day off work, a mini break or holiday

- A shopping day with friends

- A day out at a spa

- A pampering facial

- A relaxing bath

HAPPINESS THROUGH SELF-CARE

What a difference it would make if you spent time looking after yourself as well as everything else too. With our busy lives, we can often put our needs last on our to do list.

What if you could incorporate daily self-care rituals into your day? How would you feel?

You would feel content. You'd be healthier, happier, and more fulfilled. And that feeling would emanate from you and affect everyone you interacted with.

To make more time for self-care, you need to change your way of thinking and the way you consider yourself. You also need to change the way you look after yourself. What you eat, how you spend your time, and how you control your environment.

I liken this to looking after yourself the way a mother might look after her child. That means not only taking care of yourself physically by grooming, feeding, and making sure that everything else is done right, but also taking care of yourself emotionally. When you're down, a good mother will tell you not to worry and that you are great. If we treated ourselves like this and internalized that kind of affection, the world would be an easier and kinder place. You need to be kind to yourself.

SELF-CARE FOR THE SOUL

Having a daily self-care routine will help you nourish your mind, body, *and* soul.

Self-care is the greatest medicine you will ever have. Looking after yourself is of the utmost importance to help prevent disease and illness caused by stress, anxiety and depression. When you know how to get your daily dose of self-care medicine through your own *GLOW Ritual*, you can learn to heal yourself on a daily basis and have happiness and health in abundance.

This now leads us to today's *The GLOW Ritual* **for Self-Love…**

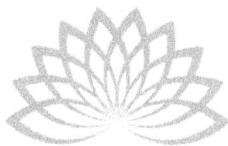

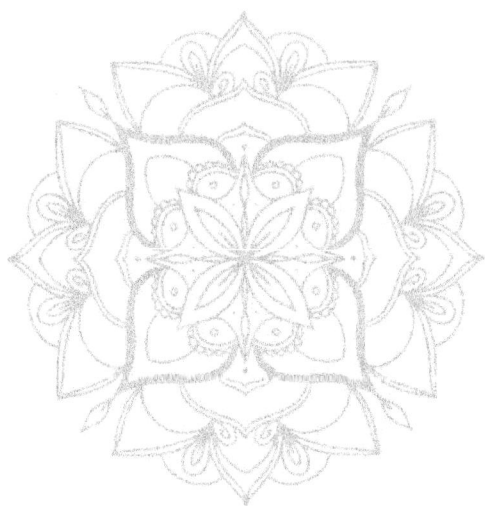

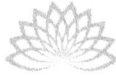

THE GLOW RITUAL
FOR SELF-LOVE

GRATITUDE & GET CREATIVE
Journaling Prompts

Today, write in your journal:

- List 7 ways you can show yourself self-care
- Try to do one of these each day of the week
- Write down how you think this would make you feel and what you will gain from doing these on a daily basis
- Write down 5 things you grateful for today

LIVE HOLISTICALLY
Life Lessons

- Making time for your own self-care is really important for your wellbeing
- You can reduce feelings of depression and sadness through a good self-care routine
- Looking after your wellbeing is of utmost importance for your health and wellbeing

ORGANISE YOUR LIFE
Get Organised

Now that you have identified ways to show yourself self-care, incorporate one of those things into each day of the week on your planner.

WELLNESS RITUALS
Time For Self-Care

Today, you have discovered how self-care is a great form of showing yourself some self-love. Pick your favourite self-care ritual and apply that to your day today.

I would love to see *The GLOW Ritual* you have decided to create for yourself today.

Don't forget to also tick each part of *The GLOW Ritual* off each day to support you in living your *Glowing Life Of Wellness*:

Gratitude & **G**et Creative
Live Holistically
Organise Your Life
Wellness Rituals

Share with me www.jaikooven.co.uk

DAY 16
A RITUAL FOR SLEEP

'In the garden of memory, in the palace of dreams…
that is where you and I shall meet.'
Lewis Carroll
Alice Through the Looking Glass

HEALTHY EVENING RITUALS

Having a relaxing evening ritual will help to bring ease to the end of your day.

Healthy evening rituals can help you restore your mind and body to achieve mental, spiritual and physical health. They allow you to create a much healthier lifestyle. You can prevent many illnesses and mental diseases through practicing Yin Yoga in the evenings and promoting inner peace and harmony through meditation. These slow movements and moments of stillness will promote calm in the body and mind.

A healthy evening ritual allows you to wind down and cleanse your mind and body from the daily events and prepare yourself for an evening of rest.

A cosy self-care evening ritual can bring us relaxing and restful sleep, which acts as a foundation for good health and a new positive day ahead.

Evening rituals play an important role in allowing you to refresh for the next day, bringing with it a whole new energy.

After a busy day, many of us wind down at night by watching films, going on our phones or watching a TV programme. However, if you do this quite close to your bedtime, it can actually keep you wired when you try to lay down to sleep. This can then result in insomnia and a restless night.

SLEEP AS A FORM OF SELF-CARE

Sleeping poorly will cause your physical appearance to deteriorate, as well as your mental health and your mood to suffer. Bad sleep causes bags under the eyes, bloodshot eyes, blotchy red skin, and the deterioration of hair, skin and nails over time. It also leads to weight gain and generally feeling sluggish because of your lack of energy.

In the short term, poor sleep will leave you with low energy and will increase stress hormones like adrenaline and cortisol. You'll feel wired, anxious, and fraught.

The solution is to sleep longer, and to sleep better! Consider this a crucial aspect of your self-care that will help you to look and feel your very best.

6 SELF-CARE TIPS FOR SLEEP

- Get at least eight hours every night – this is non-negotiable!

- Aim to go to bed at the same time each night - our bodies love predictability

- Take a relaxing bath before bed

- No technology two hours before sleep - read a book or do an evening yoga practice as your 'winding down' time

- Use a lavender pillow mist to help you drift off into a deep and restful sleep

- Instead of worrying about not getting enough sleep, focus instead on just enjoying the relaxation. The irony is that when you do this, you fall asleep much faster!

A healthy evening routine and sleep plays an important role in our daily function and can help us stay more alert and motivated for a new day.

So, this now leads us to *The GLOW Ritual* for **Sleep**…

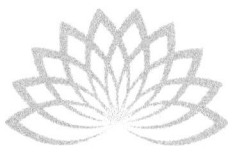

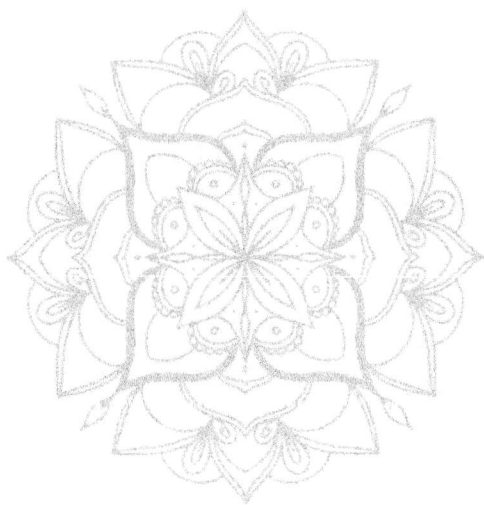

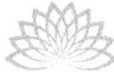

THE GLOW RITUAL
FOR SLEEP

GRATITUDE & GET CREATIVE
Journaling Prompts

Today, write in your journal:

- What does a healthy evening routine look like to you?
- What time would you like to go to bed and how much sleep would you like to have?
- Journal your thoughts and feeling before you go to bed at night, so your mind is clear of negative thoughts for the next day
- Write down 5 things you are grateful for today

LIVE HOLISTICALLY
Life Lessons

- The importance of a healthy evening routine on your wellbeing and energy
- Sleep is a great form of self-care
- Sleep plays an important part in our daily function

ORGANISE YOUR LIFE
Get Organised

Set your alarm half an hour earlier for your bedtime and see what a difference it makes to your sleep patterns and to your day. Make sure to have a digital detox at least an hour before bed, so you can relax and unwind before your drift off into a restful sleep. Make a healthy evening routine part of your daily healthy habits.

WELLNESS RITUALS
Time For Self-Care

Today, start a healthy evening routine that involves rest and relaxation. Take a relaxing bath, listen to music, have a pamper session, read a book, do a relaxing yoga or meditation class and see what a difference it makes to your evening and your sleep.

I would love to see *The GLOW Ritual* you have decided to create for yourself today.

Don't forget to also tick each part of *The GLOW Ritual* off each day to support you in living your *Glowing Life Of Wellness*:

Gratitude & **G**et Creative
Live Holistically
Organise Your Life
Wellness Rituals

Share with me www.jaikooven.co.uk

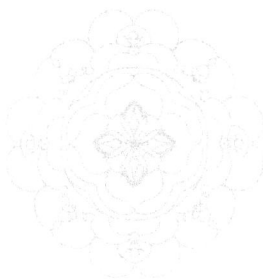

DAY 17
A RITUAL FOR NATURAL BEAUTY

*'I'm a big believer that if you focus on good skincare,
you won't need a lot of makeup.'*
Demi Moore

BEAUTY BEYOND MAKEUP

True beauty goes beyond the makeup. Feeling beautiful is different from looking beautiful. It focuses on your inner beauty rather than your outer beauty.

With my studies in holistic health and wellness, I slowly realized that it wasn't just about the benefits of eating clean – what we put on our skin mattered a lot too. Everything we absorb, from the food that we eat to the makeup and skincare that we use, has an impact.

This is when I discovered one million percent that I wanted to empower women to feel·naturally beautiful in their own skin without having to rely on fillers and Botox to give them more confidence. This included me researching for years on natural skincare and makeup, and I also have over a decade of knowledge from working in this industry.

When you embrace more natural skincare products, you feel the satisfaction of looking on the back of the product and knowing that 100% of what you put on your skin is good for you, contains natural ingredients and is not tested on animals. It is so refreshing to see just a few natural ingredients listed like argan oil and rose oil, rather than about 50 chemical ingredients that you have never heard of.

It is so much nicer when someone says to you, "Your

skin is amazing, what do you use or how do you do it?" rather than, "Where do you get your lips, or your Botox, done?" Beauty is not just skin deep. Your outer beauty is reflected by what you feed yourself internally. This is not just nourishing food but also what you read, watch on TV and your surrounding environment

I encourage you to add some natural products to your beauty rituals from time to time and see what a difference it makes to your skin.

NATURAL VS. CHEMICAL PRODUCTS

Natural skincare products are the safest and most effective means to maintain the good health of your skin.

For a long time, nature has provided the medical industry with ingredients that have powerful antibiotic, antiseptic, or anti-inflammatory properties which are turned into medicines, serums, ointments, or lotions.

Natural dermatological products are mostly found in the form of ointments or creams, which are quickly absorbed by the superficial layers of the skin. They are effective against most skin conditions and successfully treat local irritation or rashes.

The main advantage of using natural skincare products is that they are proven to be very well tolerated by the skin. This is because natural products contain no additives or preservatives and, therefore, are very safe and reliable. In addition, natural skincare products that are properly formulated to match a specific skin type are often similar in price to the synthetic option.

It is known for a fact that chemically enhanced products may harm your body by releasing malign substances into the bloodstream. In order to minimize these risks, you should consider using natural skincare products instead. They stand as a very effective and healthy alternative to all synthetic products.

However, the main disadvantage of all-natural skin care products is that they tend to lose their properties sooner; they have a shorter period of life. Unlike products that are chemically processed and contain synthetic preservatives, natural products alter more quickly, so you should always make sure to check the expiration date before buying such natural skincare products from the shelves of pharmacies or supermarkets.

Sometimes, regardless of their nature, skincare products only treat the effects of a disease, and not the factors that are causing it. Take acne, for instance. Skin acne is not always an infectious disease. It may be caused by hormonal imbalances inside the body.

Therefore, if you have a skin condition, you should pay a visit to your dermatologist first and ask for advice regarding the appropriate treatment. Natural skincare products come as an addition to the prescribed treatment, enhancing its benefits and results. Also, it is very important to check if the skincare products you choose are appropriate for your skin type before using them.

Despite their successful use among the medical branches, natural skincare products are not exclusively intended for treating skin conditions! They are also very efficient for cosmetic purposes. As a matter of fact, the cosmetic industry offers a wide range of natural products that improve the aesthetics of skin. Anti-aging skincare products are currently the most popular. Whether they are intended for preventing or reversing the natural aging process of the skin, such products are highly requested and are 'a must have', particularly among women in their mid-thirties. Anti-aging skin care products, as well as other cosmetics, satisfy the growing aesthetic needs of modern society.

Regardless of their purpose, natural skincare products are the best alternative for synthetic ones, and when properly used, their benefits are quickly noticeable.

10 WAYS TO FEEL BEAUTIFUL

Here is a list of 10 things I live by to find the beauty around me and feel my most beautiful self.

1. Smile ... It will brighten your day and others around you will feel your positive energy.

2. Stretch ... Cats know that total body stretching does wonders. Follow their example and roll up slowly out of bed and stretch gently. You can also do a Pilates or yoga class to wake up your body in a gentle way.

3. Exercise ... At least 20-minutes of any continuous activity will boost your energy level and reduce bad stressors. Any kind of movement will do, even dancing around the kitchen while cooking dinner!

4. Drink water ... No other liquid is quite like it. Clear your system. Eight glasses are recommended daily. It will also make your skin glow with good hydration.

5. Rest ... You need to take breaks during the day and sleep at night. Take breaks away from your workspace to keep fresh and focused. Make sure you are getting sufficient sleep at night since your body regenerates while you are sleeping. If you are constantly letting your mind wander, make a conscious decision to

write in your journal to declutter your mind. It is amazing how well your subconscious mind listens to your conscious mind (so be careful what you tell yourself).

6. Do good ... When you do something for someone else without expecting anything in return, you benefit in unimaginable ways. (The key is to not expect anything in return!)

7. Exchange ... Swap the money you spend on junk food for food that will enrich your body and soul. Eating healthily does not need to be expensive.

8. 'Stop and smell the roses'... Look for the good in everything. This is a tough one because most of us are trained to look for faults, errors, shortcomings, defects, etc. Begin with yourself. List all your assets (not just physical). Appreciate the person that you are and the things around you. Work on this consciously every day till it becomes a habit. There is something good about everything and everyone. Once you realise this, you will be finding good everywhere without even trying.

9. Learn ... Pick something new every day. Pick up a book or learn a new skill. Learn to do something you have always wanted to do. You can even start for free by researching online. Search the subject and start stimulating and enriching your mind today.

10. Reward yourself ... Set financial and personal goals and reward yourself for accomplishing them. This one may be something special you have always wanted to do, and not necessarily a purchase. If you have done all the above, maybe go ahead and splurge a little. You deserve it!

WONDERFUL ORGANIC COCONUT OIL

Organic coconut oil has so many lovely uses and has a huge benefit for your skin. It is also widely marketed as a superfood. It is a fantastic health and beauty product with a huge number of different uses.

Coconut oil also possesses antimicrobial properties that can protect the skin from harmful bacteria and help to treat acne.

You can pick up a jar of organic coconut oil from your local health shop and use it directly onto your skin.

Coconut oil has so many benefits and can be used as:

- Face moisturizer
- Makeup brush cleaner
- Lip balm
- Tinted lip gloss
- Body scrub
- Lip scrub
- Whitening toothpaste
- Dandruff treatment
- Body oil
- Hair mask
- Night cream
- Cuticle oil
- Stretch mark oil
- Undereye cream

HOW DOES COCONUT OIL HELP THE SKIN?

- Organic coconut oil can help with premature ageing as it contains antioxidant properties
- It can smooth the skin and keep it hydrated with a

natural glow
- It can help to retain moisture
- It can help with skin irritation and dryness due to its Vitamin E content and can also help with skin growth
- It can help you to maintain a good tan by keeping your skin moisturized after you have been in the sun

In lots of natural skincare products, you will find that organic coconut oil is the base ingredient because it lasts a long time and is good for your skin.

This now leads us to today's *The GLOW Ritual* for **Natural Beauty**…

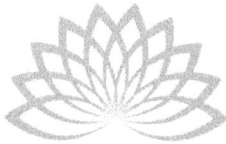

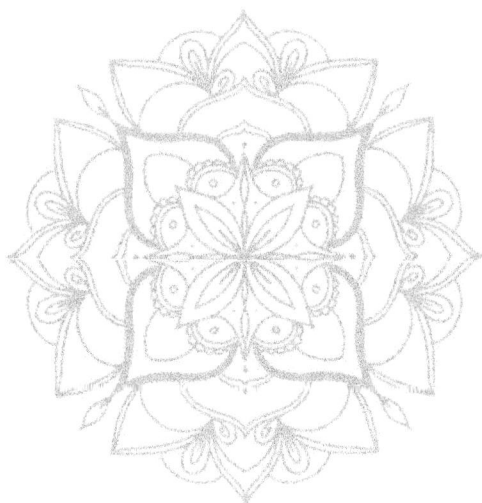

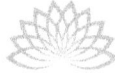

THE GLOW RITUAL
FOR NATURAL BEAUTY

GRATITUDE & GET CREATIVE
Journaling Prompts

Today, write in your journal:

- What does beauty mean to you?
- What would you like to change about your beauty regime?
- How can you do this?
- Write down 5 things you are grateful for today

LIVE HOLISTICALLY
Life Lessons

- Understand the difference in benefits between natural and chemical products
- Organic coconut oil has wonderful benefits for your skin
- Embrace different ways to look and feel beautiful every day

ORGANISE YOUR LIFE
Get Organised

Today, declutter your skincare and make-up. Look at your skincare products and observe how many chemicals you are putting on your skin each day. Ask yourself whether you are just wearing makeup to cover up your skin rather than because you want to? Maybe some of the products that you are using are causing your skin to become irritated. So, give your skin a day off from the makeup and skincare that you are using and try something different.

Make a positive change to becoming a natural beauty by eliminating any products, people, food or things that feed your mind, body *and* soul with toxic energy and chemicals. Instead, welcome new and positive things into your life that will make you glow naturally from the inside out.

WELLNESS RITUALS
Time For Self-Care

Today, make a natural face mask out of one ripe banana, ½ teaspoon of lemon juice and 1 teaspoon of coconut oil. Mash up the ripe banana, add the lemon juice and apply to a cleansed face. After 15-minutes, you can wash it off with a wet towel or cold water. Vitamin A in the banana will help to smoothen and even out your skin. Coconut oil will keep your skin moisturized, and the lemon juice will give your skin a boost of Vitamin C which is a natural antioxidant that can help with premature aging and reduce skin damage.

I would love to see *The GLOW Ritual* you have decided to create for yourself today.

Don't forget to also tick each part of *The GLOW Ritual* off each day to support you in living your *Glowing Life Of Wellness*:

Gratitude & Get Creative
Live Holistically
Organise Your Life
Wellness Rituals

Share with me www.jaikooven.co.uk

DAY 18
A RITUAL FOR RADIANT SKIN

'Glow inside and out with holistic health and wellness.'
Jai Koo-Ven

HOW TO GLOW WITH RADIANCE

When warm weather arrives, it's only natural to want to get out and enjoy the sun's glorious rays and soak up your Vitamin D. But as much as we love the look of sun-kissed skin, it's also important to protect your skin to keep it looking healthy and youthful.

Too much sun can age your skin over the years, which can appear as sunspots, wrinkles and even skin cancer.

Take into consideration these following skincare tips and you will be well on your way to enjoying all that summer has to offer whilst glowing from the inside and out.

5 STEPS TO GLOWING SKIN

1. Make sun protection part of your daily routine. It's one of the best long-term investments you'll ever make. UVA rays are strong year-round and UVB rays are more intense during mid-day, spring and summer. Wear a moisturizing sunscreen on your face year-round, preferably with an SPF of 15 or higher. Choose a natural, vitamin-enriched lotion that won't clog pores.

2. Want that summer glow without damaging your skin? A sunless tan is quick, easy and provides beautiful results. I recommend applying a sunless tanner one to two times a week, but this can vary from person

to person. If you reapply too frequently, for example every day, the results may look unnatural.

3. It is important to remember another important step in keeping your skin in tip-top shape: exfoliating. Whether it's before you apply a sunless tanner or after you've been dipping your toes in the pool, exfoliating helps produce a smoother surface and keeps your skin looking toned. Removing dead skin cells from the top layer of your skin with a scrub cleanser not only gives a smooth surface for applying a sunless tanner but also enhances the penetration of moisturizers.

4. Follow your shower or bath with an application of a moisturizer, especially after you exfoliate. Use moisturizers specifically designed for the body as they tend to have richer emollients. Spray moisturizers are particularly convenient to use on bare legs in the summer.

5. Finally, don't forget toning. Toners are an excellent way to remove residual dead skin cells, dirt, oil and makeup. In hot weather, try keeping a bottle of toner in your fridge and apply to your neck, inside your wrists and inner ankles for an immediate cooling effect.

FINDING YOUR INNER GLOW

Your inner glow is not something that can be bought; it is a feeling you get within you when you are feeling your best. I call it your daily dose of Vitamin J (Joy). When you do what brings you joy every day and find an exercise that revitalizes you, this can boost your happiness levels and make you feel amazing. This is also a great way to balance your Solar Plexus Chakra, which I talked about in Chapter 3.

That is why some people glow with health and happiness. So, no matter how many makeup companies market to you about their latest radiance-boosting products, the best radiance-boosting product is when you get your daily dose of Vitamin J through glowing health and happiness.

CRYSTALS FOR RADIANT SKIN

After cleansing your face and cleaning your crystal, you can use these crystals on your face and gently massage for a variety of different benefits.

Amber detoxifies and protects skin from radiation. It draws down positive energy and power. Skin will feel soft and relaxed.

Onyx can help with sunburn as well as fungal infections and inflammation. It helps to purify the skin and stimulates cellular regeneration.

Pink Tourmaline will help to calm and soothe the skin by maintaining moisture within it. It also promotes harmony and calms the mind.

Emerald is a wonderful high energy stone. It is the best stone for anti-ageing and repairing skin damage. It helps to reduce fine lines, rejuvenates and tones the skin and helps with wrinkles. It helps to strengthen the skin and increases the elasticity. Excess oil is also removed from the skin with this gemstone.

This now leads us to today's *The GLOW Ritual* **for Radiant Skin**…

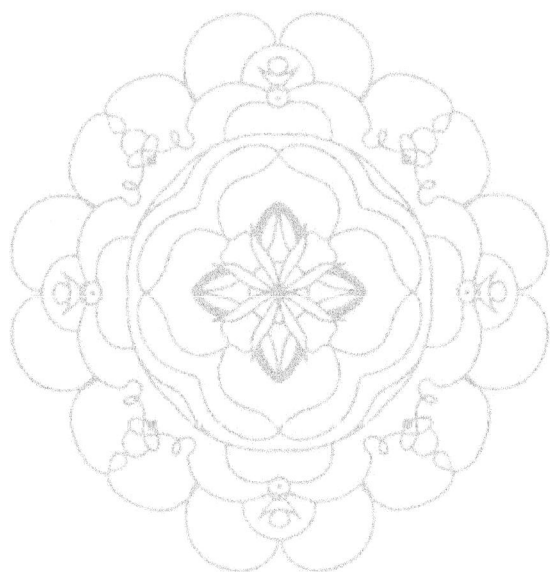

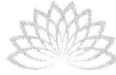

THE GLOW RITUAL
FOR RADIANT SKIN

GRATITUDE & GET CREATIVE
Journaling Prompts

Today, write in your journal:

- What things can you do to make yourself feel more radiant?
- Write down 5 things that give you an inner glow?
- What is one thing that bought joy to your day today?
- Write down 5 things you are grateful for today

LIVE HOLISTICALLY
Life Lessons

- Too much sun can age your skin over the years
- Find your joy in the little things
- Use crystals on your face to help with radiant skin
- Looking after your wellbeing will make you glow with health and happiness

ORGANISE YOUR LIFE
Get Organised

Go shopping today and get some natural ingredients to create your own face masks.

WELLNESS RITUALS
Time For Self-Care

Exfoliation is the key to radiant skin so, today, scrub away those dead skin cells to reveal beautiful looking skin on your face and body. When you regularly exfoliate, you can also help to prevent clogged pores, which will help you get less breakouts and long-term exfoliation can boost your collagen production.

I would love to see *The GLOW Ritual* you have decided to create for yourself today.

Don't forget to also tick each part of *The GLOW Ritual* off each day to support you in living your *Glowing Life Of Wellness*:

Gratitude & **G**et Creative
Live Holistically
Organise Your Life
Wellness Rituals

Share with me www.jaikooven.co.uk

THE PINK HEART CHAKRA RITUAL

In this chapter, we covered:

- *The GLOW Ritual* for Self-Love
- *The GLOW Ritual* for Sleep
- *The GLOW Ritual* for Natural Beauty
- *The GLOW Ritual* for Radiant Skin

This chapter was the building block to discovering self-love, self-care, sleep and discovering how to embrace natural beauty. We covered how to adapt your beauty regimes for radiant skin and how to show yourself self-love through daily self-care rituals. You also learned how to adapt your sleep habits for your own self-care

REFLECTION

With the knowledge that you have gained, how can you incorporate daily self-care into your life? What tips have inspired you to apply more self-care to your life?

POSITIVE CHANGE

What natural beauty tips will you now incorporate into your daily beauty regime?

CRYSTALS FOR PINK HEART CHAKRA

Pink Tourmaline

Pink tourmaline will help to calm down the skin and soothe it by maintaining moisture within the skin. It also promotes harmony and calms the mind.

Rose Quartz

Rose quartz is a gorgeous crystal with multiple benefits. One of them being that it soothes the heart with it gentle, loving and heart-focused loving energy. This crystal is great for heartbreak through a divorce, breakup or bereavement.

Amethyst

Amethyst is great to support you during the grieving process as it can help promote dreaming and work with your subconscious, so you may dream about your loved ones.

ESSENTIAL OILS FOR THE PINK HEART CHAKRA

Use an essential oil diffuser to surround yourself with a choice of one of these scents or create your own uplifting mixture.

PLEASE SEEK MEDICAL OR PROFESSIONAL ADVICE IF YOU ARE PREGNANT OR HAVE A MEDICAL CONDITION.

ESSENTIAL OILS FOR THE PINK HEART CHAKRA

Rose

This is a great essential oil for self-love. It is a very comforting and nurturing scent that supports the Heart Chakra.

Patchouli

Patchouli is great at supporting you with feelings of depression and bereavement.

Chamomile

Chamomile is a beautiful essential oil which is not only calming but uplifting too. It can also support you in having a restful sleep.

Well done on completing your fourth chapter on the Pink Heart Chakra.

What did you enjoy the most about this chapter? Let me know at www.jaikooven.co.uk and don't forget to share your daily mini rituals too.

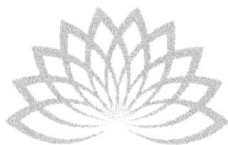

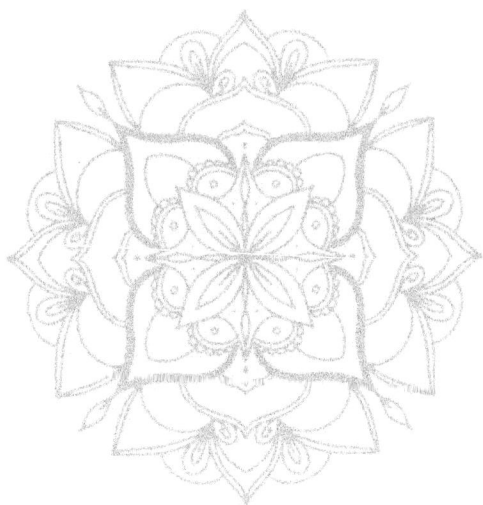

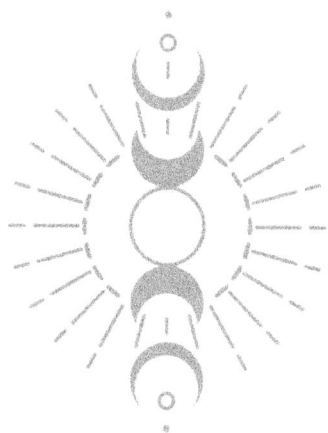

Glow with Greens

❀

CHAPTER

Five

GREEN HEART CHAKRA

THE GREEN HEART CHAKRA

The Green Heart Chakra is the masculine aspect of the Heart Chakra. This side focuses on receiving love, giving love and finding a happy balance in your life. It also focuses on bringing more serenity and calm into your life. Again, the Heart Chakra is also referred to as *Anahata* which means 'unbeaten', 'unhurt' and 'unstruck'.

WHERE IS THE GREEN HEART CHAKRA LOCATED?

The Green Heart Chakra is located in the centre of the chest, in the region of the heart.

WHAT COLOUR IS THE GREEN HEART CHAKRA?

Green.

HOW WILL I FEEL IF THIS CHAKRA IS BALANCED?

- You will be able to embrace loving energy
- You will be tolerant
- You will feel emotionally balanced
- You will have a feeling of serenity
- You will be open-hearted
- You may feel protected

HOW MIGHT I FEEL IF I AM OUT OF BALANCE?

- You may feel critical

- You may feel jealous

- You may have narcissistic behaviours

- You may be cold-hearted

- You may be extra demanding

- You may have allergies or asthma

- You may have problems with your lungs

SELF-LOVE WAYS TO GET BACK IN BALANCE

- Wear green or eat green foods which are healthy for example green peppers, cucumber, kale or spinach

- Do a Heart Chakra Yoga Classes through YouTube or through my membership programme

- Practice giving love unconditionally through volunteer work or helping a family member or friend

- Write a love letter to yourself about things that you appreciate about yourself

DAY 19
A RITUAL FOR BALANCE

*'Accept what is, let go of what was, and have faith in
what will be.'*
Buddha

THE BALANCE OF YIN AND YANG

As much as you need to take action each day, you also
need the counterbalance of time out, or you will burn out.

When you are burnt out, it can lead to exhaustion,
overwhelm and stress. You can feel like you are drowning
in your 'to do list' and everything is so consuming. I find
a lot of my clients, including myself, can feel this way
with social media. The constant noise of adverts, pictures
of people's happy lives and the fake filters can lead us to
feeling like we are not good enough and lead us down a
spiral of sadness and despair.

You can spend hours scrolling and finding yourself
farther down in the comparison tunnel where you no
longer feel good enough, rather than switching off your
app and going out into the real world and creating your
first-class life.

You can then find yourself trying to keep up with the
Jones's by working longer and harder to buy that bigger
house or fancier car, rather than taking time out to
appreciate what you have.

This is where the ancient Chinese philosophy of Yin and
Yang energies can come into play in your life. It teaches
you how to find the balance between 'being' and 'doing'
in all aspects of your life.

Yin and Yang teaches us to remain balanced between inaction and action. Yin and Yang energies are opposite from each other but are complementary. The black swirl of the Yin and Yang symbol symbolises the Yin side and the white swirl symbolises the Yang side.

Yin teaches us to slow down in our fast-paced life, live in the moment, rest and be still. This is the introvert side of our personality that allows us time for relaxation. It is feminine, with a nurturing energy, and makes us feel safe and calm.

Yang has a masculine energy that is very active and is the extrovert side of our personality, where we want to get things done. Our Yang side is what drives our ambition whereas our Yin side could be used to reflect on our next step and have moments of stillness.

(I talk more about the difference between introverts and extroverts later in this book.)

More examples of Yin and Yang are light and dark, day and night, yoga and cardio, weekday and weekend.

This is the very reason why I have a huge passion for Yin Yoga and Yin Therapy because for a long time, my energy was very Yang. I found it extremely hard to take time out as I love the work I do, so I found it difficult to switch off and just relax.

FINDING YIN WITHIN

When I discovered Yin Yoga, it was truly life changing. I really understood the connection between my body and my emotions and how I could easily release emotional blockages if I felt them arise. My time on the mat became a sacred time for me where I could move my body through a beautiful flow and get the negative chi (energy) out of my system.

I did not know what Yin Yoga was until the year 2020 when I was quite emotionally distraught about losing my stepdad. I would feel all of these emotions build up in my body and, apart from crying my eyes out, I knew of no way to channel and release the grief that I was feeling instead of holding it inside.

One day, instead of doing my usual random yoga class on YouTube, I came across a class in Yin Yoga and became curious.

Yin Yoga is different to the traditional Hatha Yoga that is a slower paced style of exercise that incorporates ancient Chinese philosophies and Taoist principles. The aim is, by stretching and holding the poses, to release any blocked chi (energy) within the body and allow for a better state of inner peace and wellbeing.

Yin Yoga helps to stretch and target the deep connective tissue between the muscles. The aim is to improve flexibility and exercise the joint and bone areas. This also helps to increase the circulation in the joints.

I remember the first time I tried Yin Yoga. I'd been holding a pose for a few minutes when suddenly, I felt really emotional and burst into tears on the floor. As soon as the whole session had finished, I felt fantastic. More mental clarity, emotionally happier and I just felt more connected. Since then, it has become a daily practice of mine and I love that I am now qualified in it and have a deeper understanding of the benefits it has on my life.

FINDING YOUR BALANCE

Vinyasa Yoga is a more active form of yoga whereas Yin

Yoga teaches self-compassion and moments of stillness. I like doing a Vinyasa Flow in the mornings to wake my body up and then a beautiful Yin Flow in the evening to settle my mind and body down ready to sleep.

I have had a lot of emotional moments when doing my Yin practice as it provides me time to observe, calm, soothe and nurture myself and understand where in my body I am holding stress and tension. I find Yin Yoga a lot like meditation; as I hold my poses, I close my eyes and breathe into those poses, and I slow my mind and body down. I feel lighter and energized after doing my Yin Yoga practice because of this.

In her beautiful book *Yin Magic*, Sarah Robinson writes:

> *Yin yoga is a time to let go of the balloon! Through Yin Yoga, we can discover a feeling of peace through letting go, and from that place, compassion and loving-kindness towards ourselves can arise. Also, in learning when to let go, we can learn when to hold on as well, reserving our strength for when holding is needed.*

Taking action and time out are both equally important in your life, like the balance of Yin and Yang energy. We cannot always be actively doing something, or we will burn out. We equally cannot remain inactive, or we become lazy and uninspired. Finding the balance of the Yin and Yang energies in your life will allow you to find your happy balance and remain perfectly present in the moment, rather than always living for the future. A good daily yoga or meditation practice will support you in finding that balance in your life.

So, this now leads us to *The GLOW Ritual* for **Balance**…

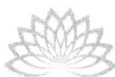

THE GLOW RITUAL
FOR BALANCE

GRATITUDE & GET CREATIVE
Journaling Prompts

Today, write in your journal:

- What is an emotion you would like to release today?
- How will you release it?
- Is your life more Yin or Yang dominant?
- How will you find your happy balance?
- Write down 5 things you are grateful for today

LIVE HOLISTICALLY
Life Lessons

- Learning to find the balance of the Yin and Yang energies in your life
- A regular daily practice of Yin Yoga will help to teach you self-compassion and find time for stillness
- Vinyasa Yoga is a more active form of yoga than Yin Yoga and is great for increasing your energy
- Taking action and taking moments to pause are both equally important in life

ORGANISE YOUR LIFE
Get Organised

Today, look at your whole life and see whether it is more Yin or Yang dominated. Organise your life so that it feels a little more balanced.

WELLNESS RITUALS
Time For Self-Care

Focus today on finding stillness and rest, or being more active, to balance out your energies. You can do this by having a run if you want to be more active or doing a meditation if you want to find stillness. How will you incorporate your balance of Yin and Yang energies into your life?

I would love to see *The GLOW Ritual* you have decided to create for yourself today.

Don't forget to also tick each part of *The GLOW Ritual* off each day to support you in living your *Glowing Life Of Wellness*:

Gratitude & **G**et Creative
Live Holistically
Organise Your Life
Wellness Rituals

Share with me www.jaikooven.co.uk

DAY 20
A RITUAL FOR OVERWHELM

'Self-control is strength. Calmness is mastery.'
Morgan Freeman

FINDING A HAPPY BALANCE

What I have noticed over the years, is that there is a connection between being overwhelmed in both work and life and the need to minimise. I realized that I wanted to be everything to everyone, and it made me feel very stressed, overwhelmed and overworked. Because of my job, I felt that I needed to know everything there was to know about everything, so that I could give my clients the best possible service. This caused me to take course after course and read a million and one books because I never felt like I knew enough.

WORK-LIFE BALANCE

It was only when I seriously knuckled down to determine what makes me happy and what I can talk about all day, that I discovered my niche. I realized that I wanted to empower busy modern women like you by helping you tap into your creativity and embrace holistic living and self-care rituals that can support you in your life.

This is when my business truly took off and I found my voice amongst the crowds of people on social media. I finally found what I felt 100% passionate about doing.

When there are too many choices in our lives, we can get overwhelmed with our decision making and then this can paralyse us and prevent us from moving forwards. Or you go the opposite way and try to be everything to everyone.

When you feel overwhelmed, just focus on the one next thing that will make a difference. You will find that the heavy weight of the overwhelm you have been carrying on your shoulders, will soon feel much lighter.

'THE ONE THING' TO BEAT OVERWHELM

In Garry Keller's book *The One Thing*, he talks about this surprisingly simple truth; we want less stress. However, we buy more things, which makes us work more, which causes more stress to make ends meet. He talks about the overwhelming number of daily emails, text messages, telephone calls and meetings that cause us to be distracted and stressed out. It all has a negative impact on our productivity levels and our health. This book really helped me to realise that you must cut through the overwhelming clutter in your brain in all areas of your life to achieve better results in less time.

Gary Keller says:

When people look back on their lives, it is the things they have not done that generate the greatest regret...People's actions may be troublesome initially; it is their inactions that plague them most with long-term feelings of regret.

Make sure, every day, you do what matters most. When you know what matters most, everything makes sense. When you don't know what matters most, anything makes sense.

We often do not listen to our bodies and think we are superhuman by doing a million things at once.

However, multi-tasking can lead to a million things left unfinished and our brains feel fried trying to tick everything off our lists.

GET IN TUNE WITH YOUR BODY

Your body speaks to you every day, but do you ever listen? It may be saying to you that you are feeling overwhelmed, tired, happy, unmotivated. Today, listen to what your body is saying and support it in what it needs currently.

TAKE IT SLOWER

In our busy modern world, everything can seem like it is going at a million miles per hour. You may be on deadline at work, so you quickly scoff down your food so you can get back to your desk. You may be a busy mum, so a quick microwave meal is a blessing when your baby is asleep. However, all these bad habits when they accumulate can cause bad health and weight gain. By changing your belief about the world, you will view it in a different way. See your food as fuel, not as a quick fix solution. Slow down and appreciate the food that you eat. When you experience more stillness in your day and practice mindful eating, you get to actually taste and enjoy the food you eat. Your body will thank you for this and digest it a lot easier. If you find yourself rushing around, slow down and make time for a few minutes of meditation in your day. Most people avoid having moments of stillness because they are fearful of just stopping to listen to what their mind and body have to say. When you step out of your typical busy routine and take a moment to yourself, you quieten the noise in your head that tells you to keep going, and you can then listen to your body's wisdom telling you to take a moment to pause.

Life would be that much easier if you loved yourself. Too many people live with low self-esteem. Too many other people are simply *indifferent* toward themselves.

What if you really loved who you were, and you were satisfied with what you had?

Simple. You'd be content. You'd be healthier, happier, and more fulfilled. And that feeling would emanate from you and affect everyone you interacted with.

How do you get from here to there?

3 STEPS TO TAKING ACTION

1. **MAGICAL MOMENTS** – Pick two moments in your day where you will stop what you are doing and take time to reflect, breathe and enjoy the moment. Be grateful for your body and mind serving you each day. What is your body telling you today?

2. **LISTEN TO YOUR BODY SIGNALS** – Have you just eaten something and then an hour later you are still hungry? Are you too full? Are you having cravings? When you make a connection between what you eat and how it makes you feel, you are able to improve your body's energy levels and mood. You are learning to tap into your inner compass so that you can listen to your body's signals. Of utmost importance is that you can tap into the mind-body connection through your dining experience.

3. **BODY LOVE** – Make the health of your mind and body a priority and it will repay you kindly. Try a new workout routine, go for a walk or try a new type of yoga.

When you take time out for your wellbeing, you are sending positive self-love messages to your body which says, "I love and honour my body and health and I will look after you." When you eat junk food, you feel like junk after. Whereas when you eat clean, you glow with health. This does not mean that you can never eat junk, but consider everything in moderation.

When you slow down to listen, it is amazing what you will hear. You reconnect with the inner voice that tells you each day what it needs and how it needs to be nourished. Be your own guide for living a healthy life of abundant health and happiness.

This now leads us to *The GLOW Ritual* **for Overwhelm**...

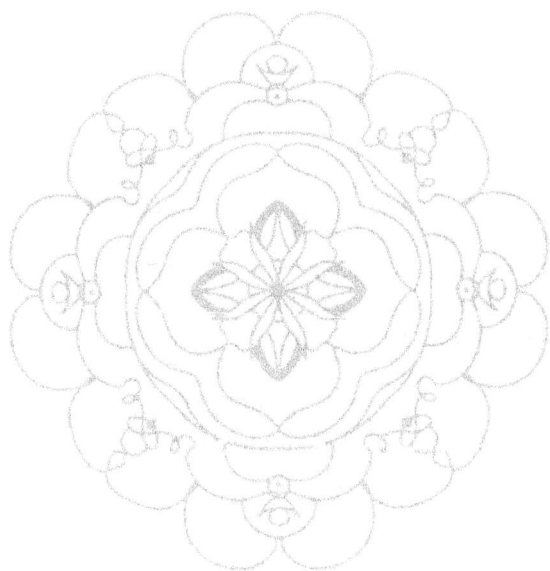

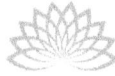

THE GLOW RITUAL
FOR OVERWHELM

GRATITUDE & GET CREATIVE
Journaling Prompts

Today, write in your journal:

- List four areas in your life that are making you feel overwhelmed
- Pick one each week to focus on completing
- How will this make you feel when you have completed these tasks?
- How can you manage your life better in the future, so you do not get overwhelmed?
- Write down 5 things you are grateful for today

LIVE HOLISTICALLY
Life Lessons

- Find your daily balance of work, rest and play
- Feeling overwhelmed? Then just pick one thing to focus on that you will complete in that day
- Get in tune with what your body needs. Does it need more sleep, or does it need to be more active?

ORGANISE YOUR LIFE
Get Organised

What in your life is making you feel overwhelmed? Look at your to-do list and pick one thing to focus on today that will make a big difference in your life when you complete it.

WELLNESS RITUALS
Time For Self-Care

Try a pilates class on YouTube or at your local gym. Pilates is great for increased muscle strength and tone and improves stabilisation in your spine to help you feel beautifully balanced.

I would love to see *The GLOW Ritual* you have decided to create for yourself today.

Don't forget to also tick each part of *The GLOW Ritual* off each day to support you in living your *Glowing Life Of Wellness*:

Gratitude & **G**et Creative
Live Holistically
Organise Your Life
Wellness Rituals

Share with me www.jaikooven.co.uk

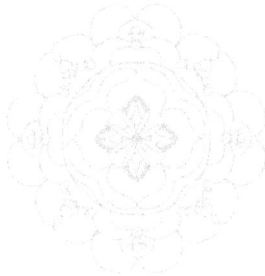

DAY 21
A RITUAL FOR MINDFUL EATING

*'A vegan diet will allow you to glow
with health and vitality.'*
Jai Koo-Ven

BEING DIFFERENT

There are millions and millions of people in this world, so why would you want to be anyone else than your own unique self?

Everybody is unique. We all have our strengths, weaknesses and goals in life that push us forwards. When it comes to being healthy, it is easy to forget that we are all unique beings and have different needs and different bodies. In your quest for the perfect body, you may assume that the latest fad diet on social media is the perfect thing for you. When I was younger, and for many years, I struggled with the yo-yo diet fad of trying lots of different things. I was not overweight, however, with magazines, celebrities and the clever use of photoshop, I thought I was fat and needed to lose weight.

So, if you have found in the past that you have been doing the same thing, don't blame yourself, because we have all been there, and there is an answer.

GOING VEGAN

To me, my life of yo-yo dieting did not change until I changed my relationship with food and changed my diet to being vegan. It was the first time in my life that I could eat in abundance and not put on any weight because I was feeding my body what it needed rather than junk food. Because the foods that I am eating are pure and not processed, I can eat in abundance, get the vitamins and nutrients I need and do not have to worry about overeating or putting on weight. My skin and body feel great and the skin on my face glows with health.

WHAT IS A VEGAN DIET?

A vegan diet or lifestyle eliminates any animal produce from the diet. This includes meat, dairy, eggs, fish and honey.

According to Healthline.com:

> *The term "vegan" was coined in 1944 by a small group of vegetarians who broke away from the Leicester Vegetarian Society in England to form the Vegan Society.*

> *They chose not to consume dairy, eggs, or any other products of animal origin, in addition to refraining from meat, as do vegetarians.*

> *The term "vegan" was chosen by combining the first and last letters of "vegetarian."*

> *Veganism is currently defined as a way of living that attempts to exclude all forms of animal exploitation and cruelty, be it from food, clothing, or any other purpose.*

A LIFESTYLE CHANGE

When I went vegan almost 10 years ago, nobody that I knew was really familiar with this lifestyle, and I would often get asked, "What do you eat?"

My answer is very simple; everything you eat, I eat, however, I create the vegan version of it. For example, if you had a chicken stir fry with egg noodles, I would have a vegetable stir-fry with rice noodles. I have learnt to adapt my diet to suit my lifestyle so that I never feel deprived in anyway. If you have a milkshake, I have a fruit smoothie.

It has become a way of life that I love, and I would never eat any other way now. I discovered so many benefits from going vegan, from reducing my seizures that I get because of having a small brain tumour to losing weight and never feeling bloated. My skin also glows with health, and I have maintained a healthy weight for years now.

Over the years, as veganism has grown more popular and restaurants have increased the options for vegans, it has become a lot easier to become vegan. However, because of this, there are many more processed vegan foods now. I prefer to eat plant-based and not processed, as processed foods can make me feel sluggish. I prefer to have fresh ingredients in my foods to boost my energy levels and give me the nutrients that I need.

QUICK & HEALTHY MINDFUL MEALS

Here are just a few meals that I like to make that are quick, easy and healthy:

- Vegetable risotto with broccoli, spinach and peas
- Healthy pitta bread pizza with peppers and mushrooms
- Exotic fruit salad
- Aubergine salad with artichokes and olives
- Banana, coconut milk and oat smoothie

Now, I am not asking you to become vegan yourself as it is a big lifestyle change. However, what I am saying is that a diet is a short-lived thing – it gives you short-term results because when you stop, you put the weight back on. What you need is not a diet but a new food lifestyle that is sustainable and where you will get consistent results.

The truth is that there is no one right diet that will work for everyone.

That is why when you take the lifestyle approach to food, it makes the whole process of eating for health a lot easier as you do not feel like you are depriving yourself, and you create a healthy way of eating around your lifestyle. By just changing one or two meals a week to a vegan or plant-based diet, you will make a positive change to your wellbeing. You can also just make healthy food swaps, so instead of a normal pizza, try making a pitta bread pizza. Instead of drinking fizzy drinks, drink smoothies or fresh fruit juice.

If you need more 1:1 support with you transition to a vegan lifestyle then I have developed wellbeing programmes that can support you in this area.

BENEFITS OF VITAMIN B12

If you do decide to become vegan, then it is important that you get a daily supplement of vitamin B12. In fact, a lot of us lack B12, so it's worth adding it even if you are a meat eater.

Healthspan.co.uk explains really clearly the importance of vitamin B12 in our diets:

It's a vital vitamin needed for a long list of bodily

functions. Vitamin B12 is necessary for the formation of red blood cells that carry oxygen and nutrients around our bodies. It's also important for your immune health, normal psychological function, and normal energy-yielding metabolism. While small amounts of vitamin B12 can be stored in the liver, deficiency is relatively common. In the UK, 6% of those under 60 years and up to 20% of those over 60 years are deficient in vitamin B12. In vegan and vegetarians, the rate of deficiency in the UK is around 11%.

As a vegan, you can take B12 vitamins, or you can get a boost of B12 in the following foods:

- Plant-based meats
- Soya or almond milk
- Tempeh
- Nori seaweed
- Cremini mushrooms
- Marmite
- Fortified cereals
- Nutritional yeast.

You need to listen to your own body's wisdom. Do you get pains and bloating in your stomach when you eat bread? Then you may be allergic to wheat or gluten. Do you break out when you drink milk? Maybe you have a dairy allergy. Your body will always show you signs in some way that something is not right.

I also recommend watching the following documentaries (many of which are on Netflix) to further understand the reason why many people are now becoming vegan. Please note that these documentaries are very graphic and upsetting, so be prepared that these won't be easy to watch:

Forks Over Knives
Cowspiracy – The Sustainability Secret
Seaspiracy
The Game Changers
What The Health
Earthlings
Maximum Tolerated Dose
Live & Let Live
Called To Rescue

UNDERSTANDING YOUR BODY

When you think of everything you learn in life, from learning to ride a bike or paint a picture, one of the things that we all struggle with is how to operate our own body system, so it functions at 100%. Our body will tell us when we are hungry, when to eat, when we are tired. You must get in tune with what your body is telling you, rather than letting your emotions run the show. A lot of the time when we put on weight, it is due to emotional eating. We are comforting ourselves with food, which is another thing that you need to be careful of as you will often feel rubbish after. Also, often when we eat, it might also be because we are thirsty rather than hungry.

Learning to get in tune with your body and the nutrients it is asking for, will allow you to create a diet that will look after your health and wellbeing and keep it full of vitality as it grows older. Incorporating healthy oils can have a great benefit too.

7 BENEFITS OF USING COCONUT OIL IN COOKING

In *The GLOW Ritual*, we have previously covered Natural Beauty and Radiant Skin and how coconut oil is a great natural beauty product for your skin and your hair. It's also a fabulous ingredient to use in cooking too.

It is a common misconception that coconut oil is bad for you. People all over the world are experiencing the health benefits of using coconut oil and it is actually one of the healthiest oils you can consume. Here are the top 7 reasons why you should use coconut oil as an alternative to other common cooking oils.

1. Coconut oil doesn't turn to fat in your body.

Unlike many other common oils, like soy (vegetable) and corn, coconut oil won't make you fat. Coconut oil contains medium-chain triglycerides (MCT), which are an easy fuel for the body to burn, without turning to fat. Most other cooking oils and fats contain long-chain triglycerides (LCT). LCTs are usually stored as fat. Since coconut oil is a MCT, it is more easily absorbed and converted to energy quicker.

People in the tropics have relied on coconuts as a traditional staple in their diet and skincare for centuries. They consume large amounts of coconut oil every day. Instead of getting fatter, it helps them stay healthy, lean and trim. When they switch from coconut oil to our modern oils, they develop obesity and the health problems that our modern society faces.

Some other people who have known this truth for a long time are those who are in the animal feed business. When livestock are fed vegetable oils, they put on weight and produce more fatty meat. When they are fed coconut oil, they become very lean.

2. Coconut oil increases your metabolism.

Not only does coconut oil convert to energy quicker in your body, it also increases your metabolism, which promotes weight loss. Because it boosts your metabolism, it helps your body burn fat more effectively.

Coconut oil may triple your calorie burn. Since coconut oil is a MCT, it is converted to energy so quickly that it creates a lot of heat. In a study published in the American Journal of Clinical Nutrition, MCTs burn three times more calories for six hours after a meal than LCTs.

Coconut oil also improves sluggish thyroids by stimulating the production of extra thyroid hormones. Most other common oils, like vegetable (soy) and corn have been shown to inhibit thyroid function.

3. Coconut oil has omega-3 fatty acids.

Most cooking oils contain omega-6 fatty acids, something we get way too much of already. Our omega-6 to omega-3 ratio should be 1:1 but it is more like 50:1. We need to drastically cut back our omega-6 oils and consume much more omega-3 oils to be healthy. Coconut oil is filled with these healthy omega-3 fatty acids.

4. Coconut oil gives you energy.

Because of the healthy omega-3 fatty acids and the fact that it increases metabolism, most people that switch to coconut oil feel a burst of added energy in their daily life.

This is because coconut oil is nature's richest source of medium-chain triglycerides (MCTs). MCTs promote thermogenesis, which increases the body's metabolism, producing energy. Many people with chronic fatigue syndrome and fibromyalgia have found that adding coconut oil to their diet was helpful to them.

5. One of the best things you can use on your skin and hair is coconut oil.

Coconut oil is one of the best things you can apply directly on your skin and hair. It gives temporary relief to skin problems like rashes. It aids in healing and restoring skin to a younger appearance. It has also been known to help with people who suffer from yeast infections in the skin, as well as many other skin problems.

Not only does it soften and smooth your skin, but coconut oil also has antioxidant properties that protect the skin from free radical damage. Coconut oil makes excellent massage oil too.

6. Coconut oil has health benefits that most other oils do not.

Evidence is mounting that coconut oil has anti-fungal, antibacterial, and antiviral effects when both consumed and used topically on the skin.

Most oils oxidize and turn rancid very quickly, causing free radical damage in our bodies. Coconut oil is not easily oxidised and does not cause harmful free radical damage, like polyunsaturated vegetable oils. Free radical damage is thought to be responsible for many ailments in our body, from arthritis to increased susceptibility to cancers.

Coconut oil also helps our bodies absorb other nutrients more effectively, such as vitamin E.

7. Coconut oil is one of the best oils you can use for cooking.

It has a higher smoke point than olive oil, which means it can take higher temperatures better. There are several healthy omega-3 oils we can choose to consume, such as olive oil, but they don't do well under the high heat we use for cooking. Coconut oil can be used in higher cooking temperatures.

It is harder for coconut oil to go rancid, unlike other cooking oils, which are usually rancid long before you even bring them home. Rancid oils cause free radical damage in the body, which is a leading cause of cancer. Coconut oil is stable for over a year at room temperature.

Because of the misinformation we have been given for years, we have lost out on the healthy benefits that coconut oil has given the people of the tropics for centuries. But now it has been rediscovered!

Coconut oil is so effective, it won't be long before we see coconut oil supplements promoted, but you can get the jump on the popular crowd and start consuming and cooking with coconut oil today!

This now leads us to today's *The GLOW Ritual* for **Mindful Eating**...

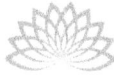

THE GLOW RITUAL
FOR MINDFUL EATING

GRATITUDE & GET CREATIVE
Journaling Prompts

Today, write in your journal:

- What would you like to improve about your diet?
- How can you do this?
- How would you like to feel?
- When would you like to feel this way?
- Write down 5 things you are grateful for today

LIVE HOLISTICALLY
Life Lessons

- Embrace being unique. It is ok to be different
- Incorporating vegan meals into your life is great for your health
- Learn to understand your body and what it is
- Create quick and easy mindful meals to great health benefits
- Create a lifestyle change that will benefit your body, mind and spirit

ORGANISE YOUR LIFE
Get Organised

The trick to getting healthy is by getting organised with your meal prep and planning the food that you want to buy. Organise your meal planning so that one day a week you can have a plant-based meal. Incorporate more fruit and vegetables into your day and notice how good it feels.

WELLNESS RITUALS
Time For Self-Care

Today, to kick start your healthy way of living. Explore how your body is feeling and look at your current diet. Incorporate a healthy meal into your day today, whether it is a delicious fruit smoothie or yummy vegetable stir fry. Make it quick, easy and delicious to keep you inspired to eat more healthily.

I would love to see *The GLOW Ritual* you have decided to create for yourself today.

Don't forget to also tick each part of *The GLOW Ritual* off each day to support you in living your *Glowing Life Of Wellness*:

Gratitude & Get Creative
Live Holistically
Organise Your Life
Wellness Rituals

Share with me www.jaikooven.co.uk

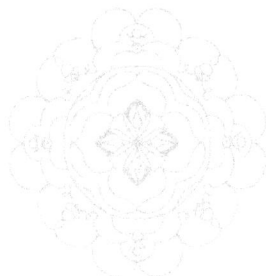

DAY 22

A RITUAL FOR MINIMALISM

'We Discovered a new life – a simple life.'
The Minimalists

FIND BALANCE WITH MINIMALISM

What is minimalism, and how can it benefit you? I am not a minimalist by any means, however, I have used minimalist principles in my life when considering what I buy. I've also seen huge benefits to my wellbeing and mental health by having fewer things. I now only keep or buy what I truly love, which helps me to keep the clutter levels down and have a beautiful, clean and tidy home. Everyone that comes to my home always says that it has a wonderful energy. This is because I keep my home clutter-free and tidy, helping the positive chi (energy) flow. When you walk into a tidy, clean home, it lifts your energy and makes you feel good. When you walk into a home that is cluttered with stuff, it can cause you to feel stressed and not welcome in that space. Even if you are not a minimalist, following a few of the guidelines can really help to lift the chi in your home and in your life, and help you on a mental and spiritual level too.

Minimalism is very personal to each person and their lifestyle. There are no set rules to follow to adopt this approach to living a simpler life. However, you should have a clear idea of what minimalism means to you in your life and what you want to achieve. This is crucial to identify because if you don't know what you are aiming for, then you will never feel like you are succeeding in your quest for less. The journey towards your goal is just as important as the goal itself. If you have a clear vision of what you want to achieve, then you can easily stay on track.

WHAT IS MINIMALISM?

Minimalism is a way of getting rid of the excess in your life, so you can concentrate on the things that are more important to you. It is a way of living that is filled only with the things you love and that align with your morals and beliefs.

Minimalism allows you to find freedom from things. Freedom from the clutter, stress and overwhelm that it can bring. It is about not basing your happiness on materialistic gains, but instead focusing on your happiness on life itself.

HOW CAN MINIMALISM HELP YOU?

Minimalism helps you remove unwanted things from your life. It allows you to live in the moment and not in the past or the future. It helps you to identify your personal life goals. You get a true taste of freedom from owning less things. Minimalists consume less and as a result spend less, so they are able to do a more rewarding job because their expenses are not so high. Minimalism allows you space to follow your dreams and helps you grow as a person. You are also able to keep and maintain a wonderful, tidy, and clutter-free home.

WHERE DID MINIMALISM COME FROM?

Minimalism is influenced by Japanese aesthetic principles and Zen philosophy. Zen philosophy places the most value on living a simple life in order to attain freedom. In the modern day, Minimalism has also become very popular by *The Minimalists*, Joshua Fields Millburn and Ryan Nicodemus, who have helped over 20 million people live meaningful lives with less, through their promotion of minimalism in the modern world.

IS MINIMALISM FOR YOU?

It is a fact that we spend around 18 hours a week cleaning and looking after our houses. Therefore, anything you can do to reduce the number of hours looking after your home, means that you can spend those valuable hours doing other enjoyable things.

Minimalist lifestyles are very popular in the younger generation as well as families. However, despite its popularity, minimalism does make people feel anxious about the changes. Would you have to live in an empty room and get rid of all your things to become a minimalist?

Here are some questions to think over before considering a minimalist lifestyle:

- How much debt do you owe? Being a minimalist makes you buy less things, so you can free up money to clear your debts.

- Do you like to clean? Having a more minimalist lifestyle allows you to have fewer things to clean.

- Are you feeling stressed? Minimalism allows you to learn how to live clutter-free both mentally and physically.

- Are you environmentally friendly? Minimalism allows you to generate less waste by reducing your impact on the environment.

- Are you feeling overwhelmed? You can feel mentally free because you are not suffocated by your stuff.

- Do you spend a lot? Minimalism may suit someone who is more frugal as much more thought goes into your purchases.

- How much value do you place on material things? Minimalists seek to fill their lives with the things they love the most and remove things with little value.

There is no right or wrong way to become a minimalist or to minimise your belongings, although there are a lot of misconceptions and assumptions.

MISCONCEPTIONS OF BEING A MINIMALIST

Here are a few misconceptions of being a minimalist:

- **Minimalism is restrictive**. People can often think that life with less things is hard when it is actually easier. You only have belongings that you love, so you spend less time organising your things and maintaining your home.

- **Minimalism means I can't spend or shop**. Minimalism encourages you to save and only buy what you truly need. Minimalism encourages you to live with less so you can let more of what you love into your life.

- **I must get rid of everything I own**. No, you do not. You only get rid of the things that you do not want and that don't add value to your life.

- **I can't have hobbies**. Yes, you can. Minimalism is about bringing joy into your life doing what you love.

- **Minimalism only focuses on physical possessions**. No, it is applied to all areas of your life from the way you eat to what you have in your wardrobe, your finances, the home you live in, etc.

Minimalism is about appreciating what you have so you can get rid of that feeling of always wanting more.

MINIMALISM AND MENTAL HEALTH

The more cluttered your home, the more stressed and depressed you can be. You may base your success on how many things you own. When you shift from materialism to minimalism, you enjoy more important things in life. You won't feel like you need to spend money to give yourself happiness. You can instead invest your new time and energy on experiences with your friends and family.

This now leads us to *The GLOW Ritual* for **Minimalism**...

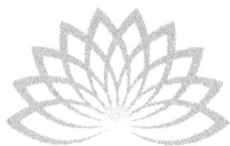

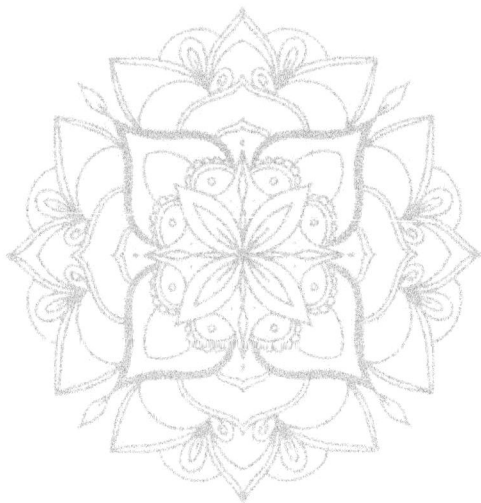

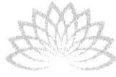

THE GLOW RITUAL
FOR MINIMALISM

GRATITUDE & GET CREATIVE
Journaling Prompts

Today, write in your journal:

* What other areas in your life would you like to minimalise?
* Write down 5 things you are grateful for today

LIVE HOLISTICALLY
Life Lessons

* Ease stress in your life by owning less
* Minimalising your life is great for your mental wellbeing
* A cluttered house leads to a cluttered mind and vice versa

ORGANISE YOUR LIFE
Get Organised

Today, take a look at your life and see what areas you could minimalise to improve your mental health. Does your home need a good declutter? Then have a good tidy and decluttering session in your home. Is your mind cluttered? Then take out your journal and write down what is bothering you. Do you have too many apps on your phone? Then have a digital declutter. Assess how much lighter you feel after adding minimalism into your life today.

WELLNESS RITUALS
Time For Self-Care

Create a new Minimalist Mantra that you will repeat to yourself daily and keep in your purse or wallet. It could be something like:

"I have everything I want and need. Do I really want this item, and will it bring joy into my life?"

This helps to shift your mindset from spontaneously buying without thinking about your purchases to becoming a conscious consumer.

I would love to see *The GLOW Ritual* you have decided to create for yourself today.

Don't forget to also tick each part of *The GLOW Ritual* off each day to support you in living your *Glowing Life Of Wellness*:

Gratitude & **G**et Creative
Live Holistically
Organise Your Life
Wellness Rituals

Share with me www.jaikooven.co.uk

THE GREEN HEART CHAKRA RITUAL

In this chapter, we covered:

- ***The GLOW Ritual*** for Balance
- ***The GLOW Ritual*** for Minimalism
- ***The GLOW Ritual*** for Overcoming Overwhelm
- ***The GLOW Ritual*** for Mindful Eating

This chapter was the building blocks to support you in finding more balance in your life through minimalising, overcoming overwhelm, creating a healthy diet and mindful eating. We covered how to adapt your lifestyle for a happier balance and how to incorporate slower ways of living such as Yin Yoga and meditation for a calmer life.

REFLECTION

When you look at your life now, is it more Yin or Yang dominant? Where in your life do you feel you need more balance?

POSITIVE CHANGES

- Incorporate healthy plant-based meals into your lifestyle each week and see how much healthier you now feel.

- Continue to have daily balance between being and doing to balance out your Yin and Yang energies in your life.

- Learn to minimalise areas of your life that are overwhelming you.

CRYSTALS FOR GREEN HEART CHAKRA

Tiger's Eye

Tiger's Eye is great for focus and determination – great if you want to take action.

Clear Quartz

Clear Quartz is wonderful for focusing the mind and bringing clarity into your life, or knowing whether you need to take action or rest.

Blue Lace Agate

Blue Lace Agate helps you to feel calm and relaxed in a hectic world.

ESSENTIAL OILS FOR THE GREEN HEART CHAKRA

Use an essential oil diffuser to surround yourself with a choice of one of these scents or create your own uplifting mixture.

PLEASE SEEK MEDICAL OR PROFESSIONAL ADVICE IF YOU ARE PREGNANT OR HAVE A MEDICAL CONDITION.

Rosemary

If you want to take action, then rosemary is said to improve your memory. It is great if you are starting a new venture or learning something new.

Lavender

Lavender is a great multi-purpose essential oil which is known for its calming and relaxing properties. If you need time to rest and retreat, this essential oil will provide you with lovely moments of calm.

Grapefruit

If you are coming out of your Yin phase and feel the need to be more energized, then grapefruit would be perfect for you as it has a beautiful and uplifting fragrance which helps to give your mind and body an energy boost.

Well done on completing your fifth chapter on the Green Heart Chakra.

What did you enjoy the most about this chapter? Let me know at www.jaikooven.co.uk and don't forget to share your daily mini rituals too.

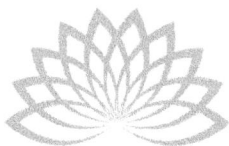

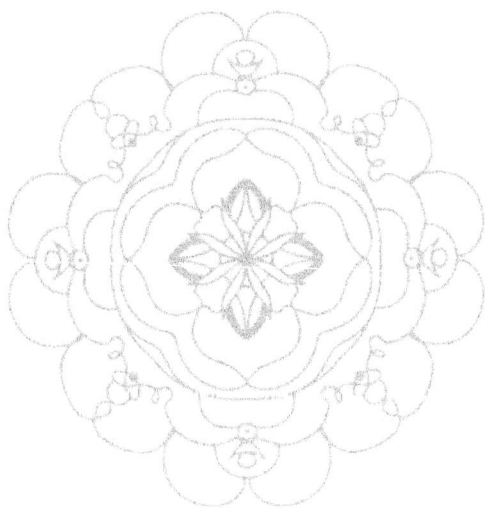

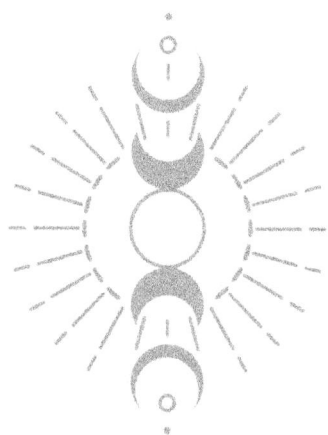

Glow with Truth

CHAPTER

Six

THROAT CHAKRA

THE THROAT CHAKRA

The Throat Chakra is about finding our voice and speaking our truth. It is also known as Vishuddha which means 'purification' or 'pure'. It allows you to be authentically you without worry of judgement. It allows us to communicate ourselves more clearly and ask for what we want in our lives.

If you are struggling to be your authentic self or honest with yourself or others, this is an indication that your Throat Chakra is out of balance.

WHERE IS THE THROAT CHAKRA LOCATED?

The Throat Chakra is located at the base of your throat.

WHAT COLOUR IS THE THROAT CHAKRA?

Blue.

HOW WILL I FEEL IF THIS CHAKRA IS BALANCED?

- You will be able to communicate clearly and clearly express yourself

- You will feel peaceful

- You will have strong self-expression

- You will speak your truth

- You will have great listening skills

HOW MIGHT I FEEL IF I AM OUT OF BALANCE?

- You may feel shy

- You may have a fear of speaking your truth

- You may struggle to listen to other people and their opinions

- You may have throat problems

- You may have an air of arrogance

- You may struggle with telling the truth

SELF-LOVE WAYS TO GET BACK IN BALANCE

- Wear blue or eat blueberries, blackberries, dragon fruit or wheatgrass

- Do a Throat Chakra Yoga or Meditation Class on YouTube or through my membership programme

- Have a daily journaling ritual where you can speak your truth

DAY 23
THE RITUAL FOR INTROVERTS & EXTROVERTS

'Quiet people have the loudest mind.'
Stephen Hawking

WHAT IS AN INTROVERT?

It was not until a few years ago that I realized that I was an introvert. I guess I always felt different, and I never knew why. I am also a very spiritually sensitive person so I find that being around certain people for long periods of time can really drain me.

I did not realise how much it had played a big role in my life and contributed to who I really am. I would often wonder why the mere mention of an office party used to fill me with dread.

If you do not know already, here is what it means to be an introvert…

Being an introvert describes a person who tends to turn inward mentally. An introvert will sometimes avoid being surrounded by large groups of people or loud people in general as they find them mentally draining. Introverts feel more energized by spending time alone or with very few people. An extrovert is the exact opposite of an introvert; an extrovert finds their energy from interacting with others as much as possible. Being an introvert or an extrovert is neither right or wrong, and you can definitely be both. To help you understand yourself better, it is important that you understand which one you mostly are. This can help very much with your day-to-day wellbeing. For example, if you found yourself feeling anxious a lot at work and do not know why, it might be because the people you are working with shout and swear a lot, and as an introverted person, this would make you feel quite unsettled.

Looking back, I was often bullied for being different and called 'boring' because I did not want to join in. I was never boring; I just took my enjoyment from watching other people be loud rather than be like that myself. I cannot explain to you what it feels like when someone bullies you when they do not understand that their extrovert ways make you feel really uncomfortable. These people may not be actual bullies, which is the worst thing. They could be your partner, family member or friend. They think what they say is just a joke and it really isn't. Simply put, their extrovert ways make you feel physically drained. They also do not realise that they are actually bullying you to be more like them, and this can cause you to feel very self-conscious and lose your confidence in who you are.

BEING VISIBLE AS AN INTROVERT

Being an introvert is why I spent years avoiding social media and not 'putting myself out there'. To me, 'likes' and 'follows' feels like being at school when you are waiting to be picked for a team and you are the last one to be picked. You stand there in hope that someone will like you or chose you and if you are not chosen then you feel really bad about yourself and embarrassed that you put yourself out there in the first place.

I feel like social media gives you that same feeling. That feeling when you post then you are secretly wishing, 'Pick me' or 'Like me,' and everyone on there is screaming for attention for different reasons.

So, as I said before, my relationship with social media is very limited because I understand the mental health damage it can cause if you are on it for too long. I do not like the feeling of 'look at me, look at me'. Constantly battling for someone to notice me and follow me. I want you to like me because of me and my contribution to the wellbeing industry, not because I post a million times a day to get you to notice me.

INTROVERT VS EXTROVERT

THE DIFFERENCE BETWEEN
INTROVERTS & EXTROVERTS

Here are a few differences between Introverts and Extroverts

Introverts		Extroverts
Energized by spending time alone	→	Energized by spending time with groups of people
Listen more	→	Talk more
Enjoy one-to-one interaction	→	Enjoy being in a group
Can feel drained by social media	→	Enjoy being on social media
More confident with people they know	→	Enjoy being the centre of attention

There are plenty of books about being an introvert or an extrovert and the differences between them, but here are some characteristics to get you started so you can understand the differences.

- An extrovert would be talkative, whereas an introvert may be quiet.

- An extrovert would be sociable, whereas an introvert may be more reserved.

- An extrovert would be outgoing, whereas an introvert may be shy.

- An extrovert would be lively, whereas an introvert would be quieter.

- An extrovert would prefer a big party, whereas an introvert would prefer a dinner party or get together with friends.

- An extrovert would be active, whereas an introvert may be quite chilled and calm.

Again, it is very similar to the Yin and Yang energies that I talk about on Day 19 – The Ritual of Balance.

THE INTROVERT LIFESTYLE

Since discovering that I am an introvert, I have found that it has also affected what exercise I do. Years ago, I would work up a sweat in a big spin class with lots of loud music, which I never enjoyed going to. Whereas now, I have my daily *GLOW Ritual* that I do at home or the gym which involves a Barre workout, Yoga or Pilates and meditation. I have tailored my *GLOW Ritual* around my personality type, and I find I now enjoy my workouts so much more and get better results this way.

In my 20s, I was definitely more extroverted, as when you are younger, you are just trying to find your way and you also have a lot more energy before you have children. However, I am now 37 with a little girl, and a lot of my introversion started when I became a mum.

I developed a quieter social life because of looking after my baby girl and life just slowed down. So, I embrace the quieter life now and I love nothing more than spending my downtime reading books or writing, looking out at my sea view or listening to an audiobook or podcast, and spending time with my family. Before the school pick up, I love meeting friends at a café for a catch up or going there to write if I am not working with clients and then spending time with my daughter once I collect her. Life is slow, it's chilled, and I like it that way. It is calm and it is peaceful, and I am surrounded by my favourite things all day every day, including my gorgeous little fluffy puppies (as I now have two). This is another reason why I prefer 1:1 sessions with my clients instead of group sessions, because I can build up amazing relationships. My clients also feel important as they have 100% of my attention, rather than them having to fight for my attention if they were in a group setting.

IDENTIFYING WHICH ONE YOU ARE

Extroverted people can also feel drained by introverted people. My calm and chilled way of life might be too sleepy for an overactive extrovert, as they have loads of energy that they need to use up. You can get extremes in both cases of introverts and extroverts.

Once you realise whether you are an extrovert or introvert, you can figure out your friendship circles and work out if you feel particularly drained by some people and energized by others. You may not realize that you are an introverted person and suffer a lot with anxiety and depression as you're surrounding yourself with extroverted things which are constantly draining your energy, and vice versa. So, it's really important to really get to know which one you are.

FINDING YOUR VOICE AS AN INTROVERT

This, I guess, is why it took me so long to finally write this book. As a very introverted person, to put my story out to the public is very hard because, as an introvert, I want to remain 'hidden'. Whereas an extrovert would enjoy all the publicity from publishing their own book and getting all the attention. However, I feel strongly that I have a message to share with you and my other readers, so I override my fear and just push myself forwards and out of my comfort zone in order to get my message out to the world.

> *"There is one person with whom introverts can always have a lively conversation, and that is ourself. An introvert's mental chatter can out-talk any daytime talk show."*
> Michaela Chung
> The Year of the Introvert

FINDING QUIET TIME AS AN EXTROVERT

If you are an extrovert, you will love being out and about or at social events. This is what makes you feel good and gives you great energy. However, for an introvert, it would drain their energy going out too much, but too much solitude can make them feel isolated.

As an extrovert, if you apply lots of rest time in between your social events, you will definitely feel a lot more balanced. You can also spend time doing more hobbies in solitude, things such as reading, writing or painting.

I think it is important to find your happy balance of your introverted and extroverted ways to live a balanced life.

THERE IS NO RIGHT WAY OR WRONG WAY

So, to sum up, extroverts prefer to focus their energy outwardly, to other people and the outside world. They get their energy from other people and get zapped of it when they are alone.

Introverts prefer to focus their energy inward and focus on their inner world. They get drained of energy being around extroverted people for too long and need time alone to recharge and reset.

So, as you are cosying up reading *The GLOW Ritual* in bed, or wherever you are, just remember that I am in the happiest place on Earth right now writing this book just for you. With my words flowing like water onto the pages of this book in your hands as we ride the waves on this wonderful self-discovery journey together.

This now leads us to *The GLOW Ritual* **for an Introverts & Extroverts**...

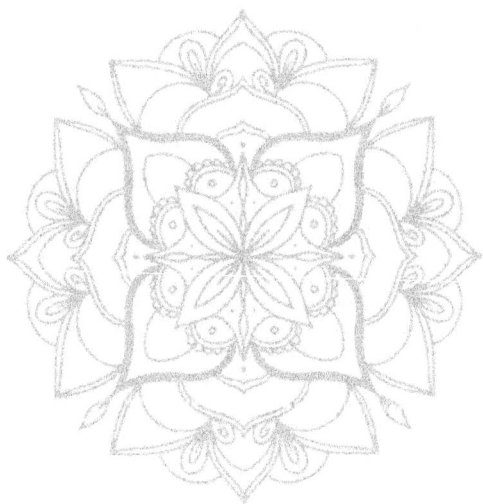

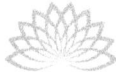

THE GLOW RITUAL FOR INTROVERTS & EXTROVERTS

GRATITUDE & GET CREATIVE
Journaling Prompts

Today, write in your journal:

- Write down 5 sides of your personality that are more introvert
- Write down 5 sides of your personality that are more extrovert
- What areas of your personality would you like to be more confident with?
- Write down 5 things you are grateful for today

LIVE HOLISTICALLY
Life Lessons

- Learn to find the balance of your introvert or extrovert personality
- It is ok to be visible as an introvert
- Identifying whether you are more introverted or extroverted can help with your happiness and wellbeing

ORGANISE YOUR LIFE
Get Organised

Today, identify whether you are more introvert or extrovert. Like with the Yin and Yang energies, sometimes you have to go slightly out of your comfort zone to bring your life back into balance. If you are an introvert, organise your schedule to go to more events and if you are an extrovert, plan more days where you can rest and spend time doing a hobby.

WELLNESS RITUALS
Time For Self-Care

If you are an introvert, today go and spend some time with friends, and if you are more extrovert, today have time for stillness or meditation and take time out on your own to recharge your batteries. Explore how this makes you feel.

I would love to see *The GLOW Ritual* you have decided to create for yourself today.

Don't forget to also tick each part of *The GLOW Ritual* off each day to support you in living your *Glowing Life Of Wellness*:

Gratitude & **G**et Creative
Live Holistically
Organise Your Life
Wellness Rituals

Share with me www.jaikooven.co.uk

DAY 24
A RITUAL FOR JOURNALING

'Write your way to wellness and release your worries.'
Jai Koo-Ven

MY JOURNEY TO JOURNALING

Journaling is one of my favourite subjects to talk about, so this section is pretty big. So, if you do not have time to read all of this today, you can do it over a week to properly digest the wonderful information that is here to support you in writing your way to wellness.

I remember getting my first notebook as a child and thinking it was the best thing ever. A special notebook that I could write stories in, draw and dream. Where my innermost secrets and thoughts were laid bare on the soft white pages. From that moment on, I felt such a pull towards anything notebook and journal-related that it is no surprise that I now have my own Self-Care Stationery range!

Journaling in my special books allowed me to express myself freely, without being judged, and I could just let my feelings flow. Whenever I felt down, my journal felt like my best friend who I could share my thoughts with in times of need. Writing for me became my oxygen and I could simply write for hours on end. This was where my passion for writing started, which in later years allowed me to use my skills to qualify as a journalist, write for magazines and become an author and book mentor.

When I was younger, I was always so excited to get a new journal; to me, it felt like a new beginning, a fresh start and a special sacred place where I could keep my thoughts and feelings safe.

To this day, journaling is a huge part of my life as I do it on a daily basis. I help support my clients to use their writing as their own wellbeing tool too or to write their own book. This also inspired me to create my Self-Care Stationery range as I wanted my clients to be able to feel the joy of owning a beautiful journal and have the inspiration you need to write for your own wellbeing.

WHAT IS JOURNALING?

Journaling is a way to express yourself through pen and paper and is the practice of writing to explore your feelings and thoughts around specific life events.

The purpose of journaling is to simply clear the clutter in your head and put it down on paper so that you can think more clearly. For people that struggle with anxiety, depression and overwhelm, this can help immensely as it can help you feel in control of your emotions and improve your mental wellbeing.

The difference between a diary and a journal is that a diary keeps a log of daily events, whereas a journal will explore your thoughts and feelings around that event, or your journal is used to write ideas down that then take shape into bigger things, e.g. planning an extension on a house, developing a new business or to project manage a book project.

Journaling is a key habit that you should encourage in your life as it has a huge number of benefits to help you grow as a person. There are no rules in journaling apart from simply writing what comes into your head and how it makes you feel.

7 BENEFITS OF JOURNALING

There are so many benefits to journaling daily. Here are just some of the benefits:

1. Helps to reduce stress

2. Helps you to cope with depression

3. Helps you to problem solve and find the triggers that make you feel upset

4. Helps you to identify negative thought patterns and behaviours

5. Helps you to gain more clarity in your life from a new perspective

6. Helps you to share your fears and figure out how to overcome them

7. Helps you to feel supported

THE IMPORTANCE OF JOURNALING

Keeping a journal on a daily basis allows you to see how far you have come in your life and problems that you were able to overcome, which can give you hope during hard times.

HOW TO START A JOURNAL

THINGS YOU WILL NEED:

- A beautiful journal
- Pretty pens or pencils
- Highlighters
- Stickers, images, photos and washi tape

The great thing about having a journal instead of a diary is that you can start at any time. Many of us always get excited for a new diary in the new year as it inspires you to have a feeling of a fresh start. Through my Self-Care Stationery range, I wanted my clients to feel a fresh start every time they turned the page and not wait for tomorrow when they can begin their new life today.

So, one of the most important parts about journaling to me is to choose a beautiful journal to write in. One that will make you feel inspired to write and not just simply a notebook that you don't really care about. You and your journal will be going on a beautiful and emotional journey together, so it is important that your journal feels special to you.

The second most important tool for journaling is a pen. As I spend hours writing, it is important that the pen feels comfortable to me and that it is not running out of ink or hard to hold. I like to have really beautiful pens as they inspire me to write and make me feel excited about writing with them. For some reason, I only use black ink pens. I have no idea why I am drawn to them, but it has always been one of my writing rituals even to this day.

Often people procrastinate with journaling or put it off for tomorrow as, like with many things, they do not know where to start or life gets in the way. The lovely thing about journaling is that no one is judging you. There is no right or wrong. You are writing to express your own emotions and inspire yourself to be a better person through your writing.

Some people can initially get a bit of 'writer's block', which is what I have been experiencing as I write this section today. Writer's block is where a writer experiences a slow-down in the creative flow of their writing and/or are unable to think of anything to write that day. Writer's block is experienced by writers, not because of their lack of talent, but because of many other factors that can contribute to their writing e.g., family issues, depression, overwhelm, tiredness, illness, etc.

For me, my puppy decided that she would be wide awake at 4am this morning, which has highly affected my tiredness and my creative flow. However, I am writing about one of my favourite things in the world, journaling, and therefore the writer's block I experienced initially is starting to ease.

Do not be worried if, when you start, you experience the same thing or at times you pick up your journal and feel like there is nothing to write. It is often in this moment that we writers produce our best work!

JOURNALING INSPIRATION

If you are lacking inspiration to get started, then try different sources, such as Instagram or Pinterest for visuals to inspire emotions or creativeness within you. Visit a café and write down what you observe whilst having a coffee. If you enjoy drawing, then art journaling is a great way to express yourself and get your creative juices flowing. Art journaling combines art of any form with expressive writing, all done in your special journal or art book, and you can learn a lot about yourself by the colours and the things that you draw.

Journaling is most effective when done daily. To start off, 20-minutes is a great amount of time as it allows us to brain dump all our thoughts and feelings so we can think with a clear head. I love to journal both morning and evening as it makes my mind clutter-free for the day ahead and allows me to clear my head of any negative emotions, thoughts or feelings before bed. Brain dumping is another form of journaling whereby you literally write down everything you are thinking about in that moment. It does not need to make sense; it can be random words, drawings, negative emotions or sentences. The only thing that matters is that it means something to you.

I often have my journal beside me next to my bed. As a creative soul, I get a lot of creative inspiration and ideas at night, so having my journal next to me allows me to write down those ideas ready for me to use the next day.

When the world feels chaotic, my journal allows me to establish order in my mind and in my life. I can express myself freely and I now see my journaling time as one of the most relaxing parts of my day; a time for me to de-stress and unwind and let my feelings flow out of me to my pen and my journal. I have my own writing ritual and I encourage you to do the same. I make a delicious herbal tea and sit in my wonderful office where I am surrounded by crystals to boost my creativity. On a sunny day, I will sit on my balcony overlooking the sea. I meditate for a few minutes to settle my thoughts and then I am ready to write away.

A SACRED SPACE FOR WRITING

It is no good trying to write somewhere where there is a lot of mess or noise. This will only act as a block for your writing and not allow your words to flow freely. You will be distracted by the noise and clutter and unable to move forward with your therapeutic writing. Therefore, I suggest that if you have no choice but to be in a messy space, that you try to clean up first. As I have mentioned before, a tidy house is a tidy mind, and a cluttered home is a cluttered mind. So, clear the mess to clear your head so you can write and do something good for your mind, body *and* soul.

JOURNALING TIPS AND TRICKS

Write Regularly

By having a regular journaling ritual, you are creating a wonderful wellbeing habit. It does not have to be for very long, but I assure you that once you start writing, you won't want to stop. Set a new journaling ritual where you plan where, when, and how you will journal as part of your day. Keep your pen and journal near you at all times so you are able to quickly and easily write down ideas, thoughts and inspiration.

Create Good Habits

In the international bestseller book *Atomic Habits* by James Clear, he talks about the tiny changes you can make in your life to get remarkable results. I have read this book four times now and it really has changed a lot about how I create habits in my life and how my habits affect my goals and the success of me achieving my aspirations.

One thing that he mentions in his book is that we need to make things simple, and we need systems, not goals. So, for example, if your journal was in a locked drawer in your shed, you would be very unlikely to use it because the steps that it would take you to go into your garden, open the lock, get out the journal and come back into the house to write would be too hard. So, your mind would resist you from wanting to journal at all because it would see it as hard work. If you want to create a good lasting habit, you need to make it easy. So, put the journal next to your bed with a pen so you can access it easily; it is the same as if you want to start running, you'd then have your gym kit ready for you in the mornings so you can put it straight on without thinking.

For example, your system could be:

After I brush my teeth, I will write in my journal in my living room.

Rather than the goal being:

Write in my journal.

Having a clear system of how, when, and where you are going to do something will make it more likely that you will achieve that end goal.

22 JOURNALING IDEAS

Here are some prompts to help you with your journaling inspiration. You can write down:

- What you are thinking
- Your problems and possible solutions
- Grief that you need to process in your head
- Things that you wish had not happened and how you can move forwards to make positive changes
- Your systems for a better life
- Things you have accomplished in your life
- All the things you are grateful for
- Your desires, dreams and hopes
- Your wish list or bucket list
- Family goals
- Quotes that inspire you
- Adventures that you have had in the past and ones you would like in the future

- Your 5-year plan
- Life lessons that you have learnt
- Business ideas and inspiration
- A letter of forgiveness
- Long term goals
- Your ideal dream day
- A happy list of your favourite things
- Confessions
- The happiest time of your life
- The dream life if money was no object

13 TYPES OF JOURNALS

There are many types of journals that you can start. Here are just a few:

- Food journal
- Travel journal
- Gratitude journal
- Exercise journal
- Writing journal
- Pregnancy journal
- Wedding journal
- Mindfulness journal
- Yoga journal
- Prayer journal
- Bullet journal
- Reflective journal
- Business goals journal

A few of these might need further explanation.

WHAT IS A BULLET JOURNAL?

A bullet journal, aka *Bujo*, is another way of journaling

using short-formed sentences, tick boxes and symbols so that you can easily categorize your entries into different topics, e.g., books to read, places to go, things to do, etc. A bullet journal acts more like a book of lists and helps you to keep a more organised life. There is no structure to the actual bullet journal itself; the writer creates what they want their bullet journal to look like visually inside. As a huge BookTuber fan (people that talk about books on YouTube), there are many BookTubers that I follow. A lot of them use a bullet journal to record the books that they have or want or to create their TBR (to be read) list for each week or month. They use drawings and pictures of books to inspire them too, so their journal becomes not just a journal but also acts a bit like a scrapbook as well, with their thoughts and feelings on each book.

WHAT IS A REFLECTIVE JOURNAL?

A reflective journal is a personal journal where you can record special moments in your life that have had a positive impact on you or changed your life for the better. You are able to see how you have grown as a person from this personal writing experience and problems that you were able to overcome.

In your reflective journal, you could write the following:

- What was the circumstance and outcome of the situation?
- What are your feelings about the situation now and how did you feel then?
- What is your assessment of that situation at this present time?
- What life lessons have you learned from this situation?
- What improvements can you make going forwards?

PROMPTS FOR REFLECTIVE JOURNALING

- How was your day today?
- What is the best thing that happened today and why?
- What are you grateful for today? (You can also have this in a gratitude journal.)
- How do you feel about the challenges you faced today?
- What can you learn about today and change for tomorrow?
- What small step have you taken towards your goal today?

BUSINESS GOALS JOURNAL

I would say that 98% of my business ideas have come to me because of my daily journaling ritual. By writing down my thoughts, feelings and ideas, it allows me to be present with my thoughts and entertain new ideas for growth. I often use my journal to keep a daily track of my goals and dreams, and this was also the inspiration behind my Daily, Weekly and Monthly Goals Planners. By physically writing and seeing your goals in front of you, you are more likely to stay on track and achieve them.

If you are using a business goal journal, then you can also add photos and make your journal more like a vision board to help you visualize your success and keep you focused. You can mind map what success means to you, how you want your business to grow and how you will create a healthy work/life balance.

I swear by mind maps, and I use them all the time. They work similarly to a spider graph where you write a subject in the middle of a page and draw a circle around it with lines drawn off the circle (like legs) to different ideas you may have, e.g., you could have a business idea about baby clothes, so you would write 'baby clothes' in the middle surrounded by a circle with the lines coming off of it with phrases like 'clothes for premature babies', 'pink clothing brand', '£5 clothes for babies', etc.

The mind map method allows your thoughts to expand onto paper and for you to see if those thoughts would provide opportunities for you and your business.

Businesses are ever evolving, therefore, this technique is one that you will do time and time again as your business grows.

Ideas that I have found useful when using my business goals journal are:

- Writing inspiring quotes
- Writing down mistakes I made in the past and how I can learn from it
- Writing about people that inspire me and how they run their business model
- What are my strengths and talents and how can I use them in my business?
- My 3-5-year business plan
- Who would I like as my ideal mentor?
- Challenges I am currently facing and how I will overcome them
- My dream business goals

I have also used my business goals journal to help me get out of an identity crisis. For many years as an introvert, I hid behind a business name because I did not want to feel 'exposed'. Over those years, I would often change my business name as it did not identify with who I was.

It was not until I used my own name that I stood proud and realized this is who I am, and this is who I stand for. So, my best words of advice in this situation are to find your niche. Find out what makes you want to get up in the morning to work all day doing something you love. It is so easy to compare yourself to others and their successes and then keep trying to change who you are to please other people. Yet, at the end of the day, you need to do this job and you need to love it. If there is no love in what you do, then you will not feel passion in doing it. It is your passion in what you do that will make a profit, so find your niche, find what makes you feel that passion, be proud for what your business stands for and don't be afraid of change. Change in life is always guaranteed, so it is important to embrace the change and see it as an opportunity to grow rather than as an obstacle in your life.

No matter which type of journaling you start to do, it is a journey to discover your true self and open doors of opportunity through therapeutic writing.

WHAT IS A MINDFULNESS JOURNAL?

When was the last time you made a drink and actually took the time to listen to the kettle whistling away or listen to the bird chirping in the morning and the simplistic joy that it brings into your life? Mindfulness is exactly that. Living in the moment and appreciating the little joys in life that are often missed.

Our lifestyles are so busy that we can often miss these moments of joy as we run from one goal to the next, doing our best to strive, thrive and survive. The constant noise of social media, family demands, financial demands, health, work and uncertainty can leave us feeling frazzled.

When you were a child, life was full of opportunities, joy and wonder. As a society, we are often told by our parents or family that we could do anything and everything we wanted in life. We would often be asked "What would you like to do when you grow up?" As a child, you would have never thought to reply "When I grow up, I am going to be a frazzled mum working all hours under the sun in a job that I hate."

Mindfulness allows us to be that child again and to see the simplest of joys in the everyday things. It allows us to slow down and observe what is not serving us in our lives and learn to let it go. It allows us to focus on what is most important to us and, rather than simply doing a job because we have to, you are able to expand your mind and discover what serves you best by slowing down and observing your everyday life.

We do not walk into a shop and say, "I want that top and I hate that other one, but I will take it anyway" so why do we choose to do this with our lives?

Mindfulness allows us to focus on what is important. It is like Marie Kondo'ing your life with keeping only what 'sparks joy'. Decluttering the unnecessary, so every moment is fulfilling our needs. This helps us to feel present and grounded and not burnt out by spinning too many wheels at one time and impressing people that do not matter.

WHAT TO WRITE IN YOUR MINDFULNESS JOURNAL?

- How are you feeling right now?
- What can you currently see, hear and feel?
- How do you currently feel about your life

situation?
- What would you like to change today for a better tomorrow?
- What is currently making you feel happy right now?
- What kind thing can you do today to make someone smile?
- What would make you happy today?
- What are you grateful for right now?
- What would you like to improve?
- What can you learn today to help you grow as a person?

A SELF-CARE JOURNAL

Now this is my speciality, especially as I created my own Self-Care Stationery range to help people just like you!

We all need to take time out of our day and check in with our wellbeing. As an International Holistic Expert, I know how important this is and the toll it can take on you when you neglect time for self-care.

A self-care journal is a journal where you record things all to do with your own self-care; things that make you happy, keep you inspired, beauty routines, self-care routines, rituals, favourite recipes and anything that means something truly special to you. This is the journal that you refer to when you are in need of a little joy and a reminder that there is plenty of good in your life. It is a reminder for the things that make you happy on your self-care days and little rituals that can lift your mood. It is a bit like a self-care spell book that works its magic when you are feeling sad.

SUMMARY

Writing your way to wellness through journaling is one of the best self-care practices that you will ever do. Your journal becomes your therapist whenever you need it. You can choose to create your new reality through journaling, not living in the past or the future, but keeping you present in the now. Each day is a new chapter with exciting new beginnings.

This now leads us to *The GLOW Ritual* **for Journaling**…

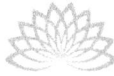

THE GLOW RITUAL FOR JOURNALING

GRATITUDE & GET CREATIVE
Journaling Prompts

Today, write in your journal:

- Ten different journaling ideas to inspire your writing
- For 10-minutes, write in a free-flow fashion anything that comes into your mind
- How can you rewrite your story in a more positive light?
- Write down 5 things you are grateful for today

LIVE HOLISTICALLY
Life Lessons

- Create a wonderful sacred space to inspire your writing
- Have a daily writing ritual so you can write your way to wellness
- Journaling is a great form of therapy and creative expression
- Journaling is a wonderful self-care practice

ORGANISE YOUR LIFE
Get Organised

Today, from what you have learnt, start your own daily journaling ritual. Organise your life to include a daily writing ritual. Which type of journaling most resonates with you?

WELLNESS RITUALS
Time For Self-Care

Today, spend 30-minutes of Stream of Consciousness writing. This term traces back to *The Principles of Psychology* which was published in 1890 by William James. Writing in a Stream of Consciousness style is a completely unedited, unplanned and unstructured way of writing that reflects your inner most feelings about your life. You don't think about what you are writing – you just write and let the words flow onto paper. It is a great way to delve deep into your inner most feelings and bring them up to the surface where you can work out a strategy on how to deal with them.

I would love to see *The GLOW Ritual* you have decided to create for yourself today.

Don't forget to also tick each part of *The GLOW Ritual* off each day to support you in living your *Glowing Life Of Wellness*:

Gratitude & Get Creative
Live Holistically
Organise Your Life
Wellness Rituals

Share with me www.jaikooven.co.uk

DAY 25
THE RITUAL OF DIVINE TIMING

'Today, I accept divine timing, I allow the pacing of the Universe to be my own. I align myself with the tempo of my life precisely as it is unfolding.'
Julia Cameron

THINGS HAPPEN FOR A REASON

Over the years, I have learnt that things happen for a reason. It may not be how we planned it, but it was meant to happen that way to lead us to a better path. Whether you believe that God, the Universe or fate is involved in this, is entirely up to you. I am completely open-minded to all religions and spirituality, and this has helped me learn a lot in my life.

TRUST IN DIVINE TIMING

'The Ritual of Divine Timing' has a path that it seems to follow with many twists and turns. You may put your ideal life on your vision board, but divine timing and intervention have other plans for you. At the time, you may feel frustrated that you have not achieved what you set out to do, and when things are not going the way you planned, this can also lead to anxiety, depression and worry. What you don't realize at the time is that your plan is just working out in a different way.

An example of this for me was when I was 21 years old. Me and my husband (then boyfriend) had been together for a few years and were renting a house. We then started getting knocks on the door every few days from debt collectors looking for our landlord who had not paid any council tax for several months and who we then found out had fled the country. I became fearful of being in the house on my own because of people knocking on our door looking for him.

This situation forced us to make a big decision to buy our first house, as we decided we no longer wanted to rent.

The day that we went to look at the house, my husband had a horrendous cold and did not really want to go, but he decided to in the end. As soon as we stepped into the house, we knew it was the one for us. Being first-time buyers, the process was quite complex going through the mortgage process, so it would take a few months to go through. As luck and divine timing would have it, the owners of the property we wanted to buy offered to rent us the house until the mortgage went through. We literally moved in within a few weeks and then eventually owned that house which allowed us to get onto the property ladder at really young age. We also benefitted from not getting caught up in a housing chain. Without the divine intervention, we may not have had the courage to buy our first home and step out of our comfort zone of renting.

THE UNIVERSE HAS A PLAN

The same goes with this book. I wanted to write a book for years and did not have the courage to put my story out to the world. Then in 2020, the most amazing opportunity came up for me to write this book and finally become a published author. My dream had come true! Since then, many amazing opportunities have come my way and many book ideas too.

I realize now that I had life lessons that I needed to learn from and things I needed to go through for this opportunity to open up for me. I also promised my stepdad before he died that I would write this book and dedicate it to him. This has allowed me to keep pushing forward with my book when it has been tough, because I made that promise and I feel that as well as writing this book for you, my readers, I am writing it for him too.

I remember reading an amazing book by bestselling author Gabrielle Bernstein, *The Universe Has Your Back*. One of my favourite quotes from her book was:

> *Get out of the way of the loving flow of the Universe. Use this prayer to realign yourself with the energy of the Universe and set the process in motion: "I step back and let the Universe lead the way.*

YOU HOLD THE KEY

Just remember that you are always holding the key to your destiny that unlocks your true potential. Life takes you on a crazy journey at times, and you sometimes get lost on your path. However, you will always eventually find your way.

When you understand divine timing and release your control over the outcomes in your life, you can be free and just let go. Work towards your goals, release the outcome and trust in divine timing. Things will always come to you at the right moment.

This now leads us to ***The GLOW Ritual*** **for Divine Timing**…

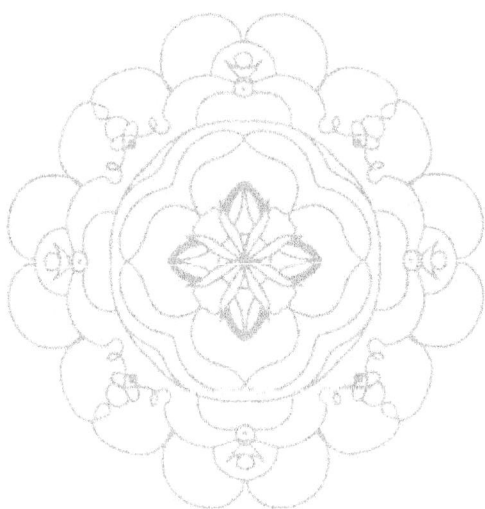

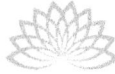

THE GLOW RITUAL
FOR DIVINE TIMING

GRATITUDE & GET CREATIVE
Journaling Prompts

Today, write in your journal:

- What is currently not going the way you planned?
- How can you change your mindset on this?
- Write 10 things you would like to achieve within the next 5 years
- What is in your control to make those happen?
- What is out of your control to make those happen?
- How can you keep making positive steps to keep moving forwards with your plans?
- Write down 5 things you are grateful for today

LIVE HOLISTICALLY
Life Lessons

- Trust that things happen for a reason
- You are always holding the key that will unlock your true potential
- The right doors will open for you at the right time
- Have a vision for what you want your life to look like, and do everything you can to achieve it

ORGANISE YOUR LIFE
Get Organised

Today, with your goals in mind, what can you change to realign with your vision and put your trust in the divine timing?

WELLNESS RITUALS
Time For Self-Care

Today, from what you have learnt, begin to trust in divine timing and control what you can control. If there is something that you want to start, like a business or a new exercise regime, take the positive steps forward to get the results that you want. Evaluate how this has made you feel.

I would love to see *The GLOW Ritual* you have decided to create for yourself today.

Don't forget to also tick each part of *The GLOW Ritual* off each day to support you in living your *Glowing Life Of Wellness*:

Gratitude & **G**et Creative
Live Holistically
Organise Your Life
Wellness Rituals

Share with me www.jaikooven.co.uk

THE THROAT CHAKRA RITUAL

In this chapter, we covered:

- *The GLOW Ritual* for Introverts & Extroverts
- *The GLOW Ritual* for Journaling
- *The GLOW Ritual* for Divine Timing

This chapter helped you to discover how to trust and speak your truth. We covered rituals of an introvert and how they are different from an extrovert, the wonderful world of journaling and how it can change your life, and how to trust in divine timing.

REFLECTION

When you look at your current life now, are you more introvert or extrovert? What journaling techniques and ideas will you use to write your way to wellness?

POSITIVE CHANGE

When you look at your current life now, how can you be more authentically you and speak and live your truth? Learn to trust more in divine timing, whilst still taking positive steps forwards each day to make progress with your goals.

CRYSTALS FOR THROAT CHAKRA

Tiger's Eye

Tiger's Eye is great for focus and determination and is helpful for writers on a self-healing journey.

Clear Quartz

Clear Quartz helps with focusing the mind and bringing clarity into your life.

Blue Lace Agate

Blue Lace Agate is beneficial for stimulating communication in your life and supporting you in feeling calm and relaxed. This crystal is wonderful in supporting you to speak your truth.

ESSENTIAL OILS FOR THE THROAT CHAKRA

Use an essential oil diffuser to surround yourself with a choice of one of these scents or create your own uplifting mixture.

PLEASE SEEK MEDICAL OR PROFESSIONAL ADVICE IF YOU ARE PREGNANT OR HAVE A MEDICAL CONDITION.

Rosemary

Rosemary essential oil is known to improve brain function and memory. So, this a great essential oil to use whilst you are cross-referencing information as it allows you to stay focused during the process.

Lavender

Lavender is a fabulous multi-purpose essential oil which is known for its calming and relaxing properties. If you are writing in your journal about something difficult or have to do public speaking, it can be quite stressful – this essential oil will help to keep you calm during this time.

Wild Orange

Wild orange essential oil is uplifting and can provide a huge amount of emotional and spiritual support which can help you manifest your desires.

Well done on completing your sixth chapter on the Throat Chakra.

What did you enjoy the most about this chapter? Let me know at www.jaikooven.co.uk and don't forget to share your daily mini rituals too.

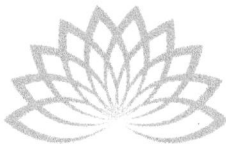

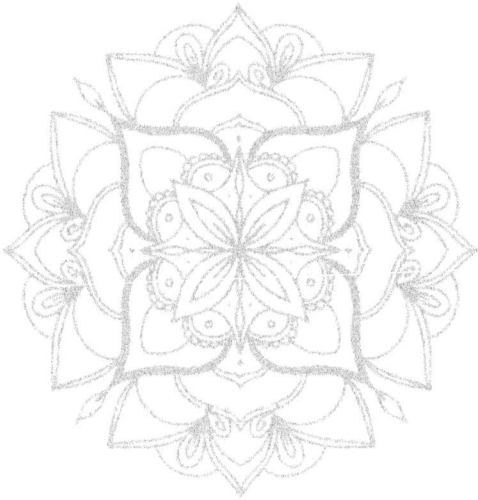

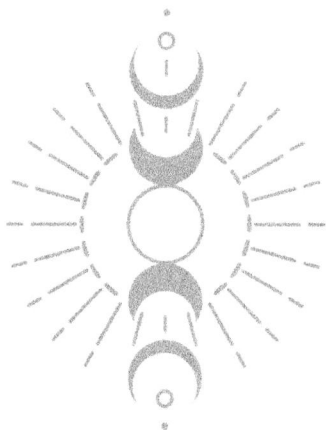

Glow with Vision

CHAPTER

Seven

THIRD EYE CHAKRA

THE THIRD EYE CHAKRA

The Third Eye Chakra is also referred to as the 'brow' or *Ajna* which means 'beyond wisdom', 'perceive' or 'command'. The Third Eye Chakra directs your awareness and how you see the world. It is your connection with your intuition and how you relate to yourself. It is your inner wisdom and helps you to keep an open mind.

The Third Eye Chakra is also very focused on your 'sixth sense' or strong intuition. It acts as your guidance to listen to your inner wisdom.

WHERE IS THE THIRD EYE CHAKRA LOCATED?

The Third Eye Chakra is located in the centre of the forehead.

WHAT COLOUR IS THE THIRD EYE CHAKRA?

Indigo.

HOW WILL I FEEL IF THIS CHAKRA IS BALANCED?

- You will feel in tune with your intuition and inner knowing
- You will feel peaceful
- You will know what you want in your life
- You will have a strong sense of inner wisdom and trust
- You may have a strong sense of creativity and focus

- You will feel motivated and want to succeed in life

HOW MIGHT I FEEL IF I AM OUT OF BALANCE?

- You may experience nightmares
- You may be indecisive
- You may suffer from depression or anxiety
- You may feel isolated
- You may lack concentration or creativity
- You may suffer from headaches
- You may live in fear of the truth

SELF-LOVE WAYS TO GET BACK IN BALANCE

- Wear indigo or eat healthy foods such as aubergines, plums or purple grapes
- Do a Third Eye Chakra Yoga or Meditation Class on YouTube or through my membership programme
- Meditate on your self-limiting beliefs and get in touch with your inner knowing

DAY 26
THE RITUAL FOR ORACLE CARDS

'You have the capacity to flow around any obstacle. This is the time to adapt.'
Colette Baron-Reid

WHAT ARE ORACLE CARDS?

I absolutely adore oracle cards and have been using them as part of my wellness and spiritual rituals for years. I remember getting my first deck and I was addicted. I loved the positive messages, guidance and comfort that they bought me.

Oracle decks are a great tool for self-growth and reflection. They can be used for spiritual guidance, but also just for fun. The messages are full of positive guidance and self-discovery, so there is nothing to fear when doing a reading. You can get many different themes of oracle cards decks from fairies to mermaids, animal spirits to angels. The list is endless.

WHY I USE ORACLE CARDS

My favourite oracle card decks are by Karen Kay and Rebecca Campbell. Karen Kay is a wonderful friend of mine who is also an award-winning author, and she is also featured in my membership programme, giving her wonderful daily guidance using her *Messages From The Mermaids* deck. I am so grateful, and it was a dream to work alongside her.

My love of oracle card decks inspired me to create my own best-selling self-care deck called *The Goddess Oracle Deck*. I designed this deck so that each day, you could choose a daily ritual for your wellbeing or positive message for that day.

For me, I use my oracle card decks every day to give me clarity and set my intentions for the day. I will pick a card and that will be my journaling and daily inspiration. Then I use my Goddess Oracle Deck as my self-care ritual for the day.

You do not need to be spiritual to use oracle cards. You just need to have an open mind to the opportunities and the messages that they may contain and apply them in a positive way to your life.

MY FAVOURITE ORACLE DECKS

Messages From the Mermaids by Karen Kay
The Enchanted Map by Colette Baron-Reid
The Goddess Oracle Deck by me, Jai Koo-Ven
*Wisdom of the Oracle b*y Colette Baron-Reid

Oracle cards are a great way to connect with your Third Eye Chakra and follow your intuition.

If you would like to find out more about *The Goddess Oracle Deck*, you can see it on my website www.jaikooven.co.uk, along with all my other products and services.

TAROT CARDS VS ORACLE CARDS

A lot of people think that oracle cards and tarot are the same thing, so I thought I would clarify what the differences are, so you can decide which would suit you better.

TAROT CARDS

- Tarot is a more structured deck and there are more rules to follow.

- There are usually around 78 cards in tarot decks, however, you may find decks with 80 or 44 cards too.

- Tarot cards have a more traditional design with a common meaning, and most decks are Rider-Waite derivatives.

- The images on a tarot deck may vary from deck to deck, however the messages pretty much stay the same.

- Tarot has a more detailed interpretation of the event.

- Tarot tells more of a story; as you turn each card, it reveals a page and together they piece together the full picture of what is going on.

- Tarot is like watching the full film unfold, revealing the good and bad in the story.

- You have to be open to hearing the good and the bad. If you are very sensitive to bad news, then tarot will not be good for you as it may sometimes trigger worry or anxiety.

ORACLE CARDS

- Oracle cards are more free-flowing and can cover many topics from spirit animals, mermaids and fairies to Chakras and affirmations. There are no set number of the amount of Oracle Cards you can have.

- Oracle cards give positive guidance and insight into

what is going on.

- With oracle cards, each card gives an overall picture of certain parts of your life or the way you may be feeling.

- In summary, oracle cards give more positive guidance and an overall picture into what is going on, a bit like a headline in a magazine or a spoiler for a film, but mostly always in a positive light. This is why many people are drawn to them.

With this knowledge, which do you think would be right for you?

So, this now leads us to *The GLOW Ritual* **for Oracle Cards**...

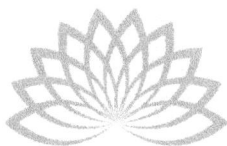

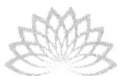

THE GLOW RITUAL
FOR ORACLE CARDS

GRATITUDE & GET CREATIVE
Journaling Prompts

Today, write in your journal:

- If you have any card decks, pick a card and journal about your thoughts and feelings about that card
- Journal about how you can learn to trust your intuition better
- What is your inner wisdom guiding you to do?
- Write down 5 things you are grateful for today

LIVE HOLISTICALLY
Life Lessons

- Oracle cards and tarot cards are a fantastic form of spiritual guidance
- Be open to the opportunities and spiritual messages that you receive
- Oracle cards and tarot cards are great to use to set positive intentions

ORGANISE YOUR LIFE
Get Organised

Organise time in each day to reflect and reset. Use spiritual tools such as oracle cards or journaling to help you to organise time just for you.

WELLNESS RITUALS
Time For Self-Care

Today, either explore oracle cards or tarot cards in more detail, if this is something that you are interested in, or spend some time in meditation to connect with your intuition.

I would love to see *The GLOW Ritual* you have decided to create for yourself today.

Don't forget to also tick each part of *The GLOW Ritual* off each day to support you in living your *Glowing Life Of Wellness*:

Gratitude & **G**et Creative
Live Holistically
Organise Your Life
Wellness Rituals

Share with me www.jaikooven.co.uk

DAY 27
A RITUAL FOR THE LAW OF ATTRACTION

'Ask for what you want and be prepared to get it.'
Maya Angelou

WHAT IS THE LAW OF ATTRACTION?

In the New Thought philosophy, the Law of Attraction is the belief that positive or negative thoughts bring positive or negative experiences. The belief is that thoughts are made of 'pure energy', so like attracts like. For example, if you think you are going to have a bad day, you will attract bad things in your day.

The Law of Attraction is a great philosophy to use to combine cognitive reframing techniques, affirmations and creative visualizations like vision boards to allow more positive things to come into your life. Think of yourself as a magnet: what you put out, you attract. That is The Law of Attraction. If you are a negative person, you will attract negativity into your life.

I have used Law of Attraction techniques in my life for years and it never ceases to amaze me how it really does change your life and perspective. If bad things happen to me now, rather than feeding the negativity, I just know that it needed to happen for better things to come.

LIKE ATTRACTS LIKE

When you book a luxury holiday, you plan everything out, from the time that you are leaving to the clothes that you want to wear, where you are going to eat, your spending money and where you are going to stay. This is you creating your first-class life for the holiday that you want to create.

The Law of Attraction works in the same way. You tell the Universe what you want and then live-in alignment with that goal and vision.

ASK, ALIGN YOURSELF, BELIEVE AND RECEIVE

The Law of Attraction works in the same way as planning your dream luxury holiday, however, you are applying it to your life. What do I want in life? Where do I want to go? Who do I want to go with? What job do I want to do? What do I need to learn to get to where I want to go? It is your own map that you use to create the masterpiece that is your life and every day, you live in alignment with the masterpiece that you want to create.

The Law of Attraction describes a phenomenon where what you believe to be true can actually become a reality, simply because you actually believe it, and you live in alignment for the reality you want to create for yourself.

As you are probably aware, you tend to like things that you do well in, and so by thinking you're good at something, you will then start to enjoy it more, and put in more time as a result. This is the reason why sports psychologists use the 'sandwich' technique when giving criticism - positive, negative, positive.

This way, they can give their advice without damaging the esteem of the sprinter or gymnast. Therefore, you need to try and constantly increase your own self-esteem and closely control how you perceive yourself to increase your success and believe that you can achieve anything you want in life.

DISCOVERING *THE SECRET*

The Secret is a very famous self-help book by Rhonda Byrne which was also made into a film. It is based on the belief of the Law of Attraction

I have touched on a lot of the Law of Attraction techniques in this book, however, if you want to delve deeper, I would definitely recommend reading this book. Rhonda explains the Law of Attraction in greater detail and how it can really change your life. It is such an inspirational book with some great insights from some amazing spiritual leaders. It is the book that introduced me to the Law of Attraction and helped to change my life.

> *"Decide what you want. Believe you can have it. Believe you deserve it and believe it's possible for you. And then close your eyes every day for several minutes, and visualize having what you already want, feeling the feelings of already having it. Come out of that and focus on what you're grateful for already, and really enjoy it. Then go into your day and release it to the Universe and trust that the Universe will figure out how to manifest it."*
> *Jack Canfield*
> *The Secret*

THE LAW OF ATTRACTION AND YOU

How you perceive yourself speaks volumes to other people and you will reveal your self-confidence in subtle ways – the way you walk, the way you speak, the way you dress and the way you act.

If you act as though you deserve respect, then you'll start to believe it yourself, and if you start to believe in yourself, then so will others.

This goes deeper than abstract opinions and can even be used to generate wealth and success. For example, you may have heard of the term 'dress for success' or 'power dressing'. By dressing well, you feel good, which gives you the confidence to go after your goals and eventually achieve them. If you project an image of being wealthy, then others will begin to think you're rich and successful. This can mean that your boss is more likely to give you a promotion (hence the saying "you should dress for the job you want, not the job you're in"). It also means others will be more likely to trust you in business and that other wealthy people will gravitate towards you. You become a magnet for success and successful people.

So, dressing well can make others believe you are successful and can make you feel successful, too. Although, you can't just look the part, you must act the part and feel the part. Over time, by mimicking the actions and behaviour of someone successful, you will start to pick them up as habits. These daily habits help you stay in alignment with your goals and put out to the Universe that you are serious about your intentions. When you believe anything is possible, the magic happens, and the Universe opens the doors of opportunities for you.

> *"What you think, you become.*
> *What you feel, you attract.*
> *What you imagine, you create."*
> *Buddha*

This now leads us to today's ***The GLOW Ritual*** **for The Law of Attraction**…

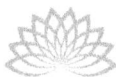

THE GLOW RITUAL
FOR THE LAW OF ATTRACTION

GRATITUDE & GET CREATIVE
Journaling Prompts

Today, write in your journal:

- List 5 things in your life that you want to attract
- How can you stay in alignment to receive what you have asked for?
- What are the positive steps you can take towards achieving your goals?
- Write down 5 things you are grateful for today

LIVE HOLISTICALLY
Life Lessons

- When you believe anything is possible, the magic happens
- The Law of Attraction describes a phenomenon where what you believe to be true can actually become your reality, simply because you believe it - you live in alignment with the reality you want to create for yourself

ORGANISE YOUR LIFE
Get Organised

Today, you are going to practice the Law of Attraction in an enjoyable way by acting all day as if you are living the life of your dreams. What will you wear? Where would you go? What would you attract in your life? What does it feel like to do your dream job? Reflect on how it feels to live your dream life today.

WELLNESS RITUALS
Time For Self-Care

Start a Morning Manifesting Routine that will set your day up for success. A great morning routine has a lot of health benefits for your mind and body, and it also makes your day more productive. So, plan your day out for success with writing rituals, workouts, healthy eating, mindfulness and goals that you want to achieve for today.

I would love to see *The GLOW Ritual* you have decided to create for yourself today.

Don't forget to also tick each part of *The GLOW Ritual* off each day to support you in living your *Glowing Life Of Wellness*:

Gratitude & **G**et Creative
Live Holistically
Organise Your Life
Wellness Rituals

Share with me www.jaikooven.co.uk

DAY 28
THE RITUAL OF VISION BOARDS

'What you surround yourself with, you become.'
Jai Koo-Ven

THE POWER OF VISUALIZATION

Imagine a beautiful beach with gorgeous sounds of the relaxing waves and the sun shining down on your face as you relax on the soft sand. How does this make you feel? This is the power of visualization. The ability to create images in your mind's eye of the life that you want.

The problem is that many of us go about our day-to-day lives focusing on what we don't want or worrying about the 'what ifs'. Again, this is another form of the Law of Attraction; what you focus on becomes your reality. You are a magnet for what you want to attract in your life.

Visualization is not about being an inactive dreamer who is just hoping that someday their life will get better. Visualization is about visualizing the result you want to attract in your life. This is how many athletes all over the world excel in sports because they visualize winning; the feeling they will get when they score that goal or cross that finishing line and they condition their mind for success.

> *"As a kid, I always idolized the winning athletes. It is one thing to idolize heroes. It is quite another to visualize yourself in their place. When I saw great people, I said to myself: I can be there."*
> *Arnold Schwarzenegger*

WHEN I SEE IT, I WILL BELIEVE IT

You can visualize through meditation or journaling to attract the outcome that you want.

Here is a 4-step visualization process to help you get started

1. KNOW WHAT YOU WANT

Again, like the Law of Attraction, if you do not know what you want, then how will you know what to attract, visualize or ask for? You need to understand why you want what you have asked for in order to manifest it into your life. This is easily achieved by doing some mindset work on what you value in your life and what brings you the most joy.

2. HAVE A VISION

Create a clear vision for what you want to manifest in your life. You can write this down in detail through journaling or create a vision board. This will help you create a visual picture of what you want, which you can use daily as a reminder.

3. CREATE THE EMOTION

Once you have created the vision, it is now time to tune into the emotion that surrounds your vision. What will it feel like when you achieve that goal? Do not get caught up in all the different steps that you would need to do to get there at this stage, just focus on the feeling. Then, once you have mastered that, you start your masterplan by setting daily, weekly and monthly goals to get you the results that you want.

4. BE PATIENT & TAKE DAILY ACTION

Things take time, and 'quick fix' solutions will never give you the lasting results that you require. Creating your dream life will take time and it won't just happen overnight. However, step by step, day by day, with consistent action, you will achieve your goal. Don't focus on how far you have to go, just focus on what you can do right now, enjoying the process and being present.

In my chapter about 'A Ritual for Taking Action' and Time Out, I talked about how I achieved a huge amount in one year during a global pandemic. Visualization was my number one practice I did every day to achieve those goals. I knew 100% that I could achieve everything I wanted in that year by using visualization and Law of Attraction techniques to make it my reality.

> *"Nothing is impossible. The word itself*
> *says, I am possible."*
> *Audrey Hepburn*

CREATING A VISION BOARD

You never travel without knowing the destination that you are trying to reach. Your goals are the same thing. How do you know how you are going to achieve your goals if you do not know your final destination?

HOW TO IDENTIFY YOUR GOALS AND WHAT MATTERS TO YOU

One of my favourite things to do when I want to feel inspired is to create mind maps of my plans. It allows me to be able to put all my jumbled thoughts onto paper and plan a way forward.

HOW TO CREATE A MIND MAP

I have spoken about mind maps earlier on in this book, however, this is another way of drawing one…

Get a plain piece of paper, and in the middle of it write the word 'GOALS' with a circle around it. From that, draw lines like a spider with different headings such as 'Personal', 'Business', 'Health', 'Life' and 'Family'. You can use different coloured pens, drawings and images to also inspire you. Mind maps are similar to spider diagrams although the difference between the two is that spider diagrams do not always use colour and are not as structured as mind maps with no specific rules.

Once you have created your mind map, under the headings you can write what goal you would like to achieve and when you would like to achieve it by. If you prefer a more artistic way of doing a mind map, then create a vision board instead. So, instead of writing what you want to achieve, you can stick inspiring photos on a pin board, or create a digital version using Pinterest instead.

The reason why the mind map and vision boards are so effective is because they allow you to plan towards your goals when you can clearly visualize them. This can help you remain focused, positive and motivated with what you want to achieve. I review my goals daily and if I ever feel overwhelmed by them then I just ask myself "What is the next thing that will make a difference?"

Have fun creating your vision boards to inspire you to create the life you want. Remember that anything is possible if you have a plan on how you will get there.

This now leads us to *The GLOW Ritual* for **Vision Boards**…

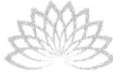

THE GLOW RITUAL
FOR VISION BOARDS

GRATITUDE & GET CREATIVE
Journaling Prompts

Today, write in your journal:

- Write down everything that you want in life
- Create mind maps on how you will achieve those goals and when
- Reflect on how it would feel for you to achieve all your goals
- Write down 5 things you are grateful for today

LIVE HOLISTICALLY
Life Lessons

- Visualization is a great way to manifest the life that you want
- Vision boards allow you to turn your dream into a physical object By seeing what you want, you are more likely to be able to achieve it
- Your vision board acts as the road map of your dream destination

ORGANISE YOUR LIFE
Get Organised

Cut out pictures from magazines or print out pictures on the internet that inspire you and organise them into these categories: Work, Life, Family, Money, Health & Home ready for today's Wellness Rituals.

WELLNESS RITUALS
Time For Self-Care

Today, have a fun day creating your own vision board or mind map to inspire you to achieve your goals. You can create a digital one, however, you will energetically connect better with one that you have made by hand. Make a habit of looking at it regularly to inspire you each day.

I would love to see *The GLOW Ritual* you have decided to create for yourself today.

Don't forget to also tick each part of *The GLOW Ritual* off each day to support you in living your *Glowing Life Of Wellness*:

Gratitude & **G**et Creative
Live Holistically
Organise Your Life
Wellness Rituals

Share with me www.jaikooven.co.uk

THE THIRD EYE CHAKRA RITUAL

In this chapter, we covered:

- *The GLOW Ritual* for Oracle Cards
- *The GLOW Ritual* for The Law of Attraction
- *The GLOW Ritual* for Vision Boards

This chapter supported you in learning to follow your intuition and listen to your inner wisdom. We covered what oracle cards are and the difference between oracle cards and tarot cards and how you can use them for guidance. You learnt about the Law of Attraction and how you can attract everything you want into your life through living in alignment with what you want. We also explored the power of vision boards to manifest the life you want.

REFLECTION

When you look at your vision board, how different is the life you have now to the life that you want? How will you stay in alignment in pursuit of your goals?

POSITIVE CHANGE

Practising the Law of Attraction and visualization daily is life-changing and can really inspire you to believe that anything is possible. Simply ask, align yourself with your goals, believe and receive, and stay in alignment for what you have asked for.

CRYSTALS FOR THIRD EYE CHAKRA

Lapis Lazuli

This crystal looks so beautiful with its gorgeous blue hue. It helps to block negative energy and allows positivity to flow to you.

Clear Quartz

Clear Quartz is great at focusing the mind and bringing clarity into your life.

Snowflake Obsidian

This crystal is calming and soothing, providing peace and balance in the mind, body *and* spirit. It recognizes your uniqueness and your individuality. It will remove feelings of isolation if you are alone, allowing you to remain confident and secure and encouraging you to be your true self.

ESSENTIAL OILS FOR THE THIRD EYE CHAKRA

Use an essential oil diffuser to surround yourself with a choice of one of these scents or create your own uplifting mixture.

PLEASE SEEK MEDICAL OR PROFESSIONAL ADVICE IF YOU ARE PREGNANT OR HAVE A MEDICAL CONDITION.

Frankincense

Frankincense is the perfect essential oil for calming and soothing the mind, body and spirit. It is a nurturing oil that allows us to gain creative clarity.

Basil

Basil is great for stimulating, calming, energizing, clarifying and uplifting the mind. It can also soothe headaches and eliminate odour-causing bacteria, as well as repel insects.

Fennel

Fennel is wonderful for supporting you both spiritually and emotionally. It can help with motivation, self-confidence and can support you in living an authentic life in line with your values.

Well done on completing your seventh chapter on the Third Eye Chakra.

What did you enjoy the most about this chapter? Let me know at www.jaikooven.co.uk and don't forget to share your daily mini rituals too.

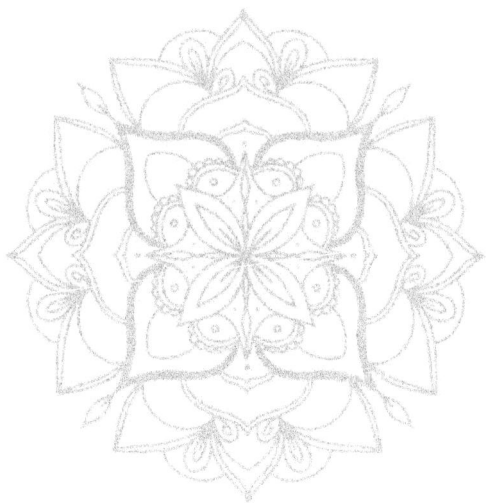

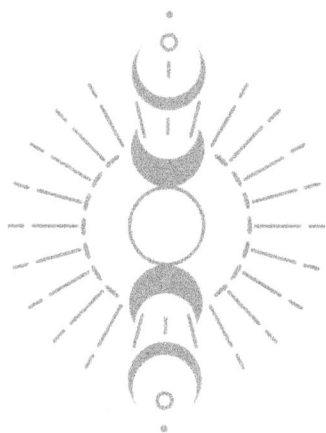

Glow with Wisdom

❧

CHAPTER

Eight

CROWN CHAKRA

THE CROWN CHAKRA

The Crown Chakra connects us to our spirituality which essentially means 'the spiritual self'. It is also referred to as Sahasrara which means 'thousand petal lotus' and represents the divine lotus. The Crown Chakra is like the opening of a lotus to the sun and world around it.

The Crown Chakra is the unity and interconnectedness of all things. It connects us to our higher self and makes us feel at one with the Universe.

WHERE IS THE CROWN CHAKRA LOCATED?

The Crown Chakra is located at the top of the head.

WHAT COLOUR IS THE CROWN CHAKRA?

Violet.

HOW WILL I FEEL IF THIS CHAKRA IS BALANCED?

- You will feel in tune with your intuition and inner knowing
- You will feel peaceful
- You will know what you want in your life
- You will feel in tune with your spiritual side
- You will feel blessed for your spiritual connection
- You will feel open-minded and connected to the Universe
- You will have a strong nervous system

HOW MIGHT I FEEL IF I AM OUT OF BALANCE?

- You may suffer from mental health issues
- You may feel fear
- You may have memory or learning problems
- You may be in spiritual crisis
- You may lack concentration or creativity
- You may suffer from headaches
- You may live in fear of the truth
- You may feel broken with a lack of apathy
- You may be materialistic

SELF-LOVE WAYS TO GET BACK IN BALANCE

- Wear violet
- Do a Crown Chakra Yoga or Meditation Class on YouTube or through my membership programme
- Get a clear quartz crystal which is known as the 'The Master Healer', as it is the crystal of power and amplifies energy

DAY 29
A RITUAL FOR CALM

'There is peace even in the storm.'
Vincent Van Gogh

CREATING CALM IN CHAOS

Let's be honest, life is chaotic, no matter whether you are a busy entrepreneur, stay-at-home mum, go out to work or are a housewife. No matter what you do, in life nowadays everything goes a million miles an hour with no time to fit everything all in and no time to breathe. We are connected 24/7 to news, shops, emails and social media, and it is exhausting.

Working for myself, I can easily get caught in this loop and recently found myself so exhausted my brain and body just told me to stop. I would not feel guilty about taking time out if I worked for another company, yet I kept pushing and pushing myself because I work for myself. I had so many projects on that I wanted to complete, that I felt I could not have a break.

Everything just felt so chaotic and out of control and knew I needed to do something different to get better results. So, I booked a week off to reset and journaled about the dream life that I would want to live and not the chaos that I had created.

People often assume that spiritual gurus, entrepreneurs, mentors, coaches and housewives with the perfect clean house have it all together. This could not be further from the truth. We have all been through the pain, trauma and chaos. However, rather than dig an early grave and hop in, we pursue a way forward. We see the light in every dark cloud and know that there is a way out; we just need to learn from our mistakes and find another way.

FINDING SERENITY IN STILLNESS

This week, I stopped running on the treadmill or trying to be of service to others, and I figured out my own ways of filling my own cup up and taking some time out to reflect, reset and move forward.

It is hard when you have a creative brain with so many ideas and you know that you are here to support others. All you want to do is help and be of service, but in doing so, your cup goes empty and at times you may have nothing left to give. The problem with society and social media nowadays is that you are bombarded with information so much that you don't know what your own thoughts are half the time. You are being sold to, told you are not enough if you don't own this, you're a failure if you don't get a degree or do this course, you are rubbish and unlikeable if you don't have a lot of followers on social media - this constant noise is enough to make anybody doubt themselves and their abilities and make your mind feel in chaos.

RESET YOUR MINDSET

This week I invite you to find or create calm in the chaos of your busy life. To keep your feet firmly on the ground and remain unshakable to the life around you.

You must hit a point like this sometimes where you just need to take a step back and see your life from a different view. Time out to reset, reflect and make positive changes. If you carry on doing the same things all the time, you will get the same results. You will think you are invincible, unstoppable and you have everything under control, until you crash and burn.

So, I encourage you to reflect on your life today. Are you living the life you want to live or are you just running on the same hamster wheel again and again and getting nowhere? Are you feeling exhausted or energized? Are you living your life with purpose

My reset week is allowing me to reset all areas in my life and shape them to how I want them to look. It is allowing me to make time for my own self-care first before I serve others.

Especially in what I do, you are always giving positive energy out, so it is important that you have some positive energy for yourself too, so that you can strive and thrive in life.

ESTABLISH YOUR BASELINE FOR BALANCE

My reset week will consist of getting my house and brain in order and decluttering any negative thoughts. Releasing and letting go with daily rejuvenating yoga flows and finding moments of stillness with meditation, reading and reflection. Having walks on the beach and daily self-care rituals of pampering. Spending time out in nature as I ground myself once again and, of course, writing my way to wellness.

Looking after your wellness is an endless journey. You are constantly having to adapt and change to make life flow for you. You are constantly having to rebalance yourself one way or another.

EVEN THE MOST PERFECT GEMS ARE FLAWED

Life is not perfect. This pressure of 'the perfect life' can leave us feeling exhausted and chasing an endless dream. This is why the balance of healthy Yin and Yang energies in your life are so important; the balance of 'being' and 'doing'.

Having daily wellness rituals will always bring you back into balance whenever life gets hard. As you tune into your wellbeing and realise that it's time to make a change, you can invite calm back into your life once again.

This now leads us to *The GLOW Ritual* **for Calm**…

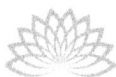

THE GLOW RITUAL
FOR CALM

GRATITUDE & GET CREATIVE
Journaling Prompts

Today, write in your journal:

- Write down 5 things that will make your days feel calmer
- Pick one to focus on and write down why this matters to you
- What can you do to make this scenario calmer for you?
- Write down 5 things that you are grateful for today.

LIVE HOLISTICALLY
Life Lessons

- Life is not perfect, and it is important to remember that even the most perfect gems are flawed
- Finding daily serenity in stillness
- Looking after your wellness is an endless journey
- Establish your baseline for balance

ORGANISE YOUR LIFE
Get Organised

Today, create calm in your day by taking time to declutter your mindset of negative thoughts through journaling, meditation, or physically decluttering your space for 20-minutes.

WELLNESS RITUALS
Time For Self-Care

Create a calm space in your home or garden that you can retreat to whenever you need it – your own special sacred space filled with your favourite things that inspire you. This can then become your special place that you visit daily for quiet time, meditation, yoga or reading.

I would love to see *The GLOW Ritual* you have decided to create for yourself today.

Don't forget to also tick each part of *The GLOW Ritual* off each day to support you in living your *Glowing Life Of Wellness*:

Gratitude & **G**et Creative
Live Holistically
Organise Your Life
Wellness Rituals

Share with me www.jaikooven.co.uk

DAY 30
THE RITUAL OF CONTENTMENT

'Our treasure is not outside us.
It's not something we swim towards; we already have
it.'
Colette Baron-Reid

OPEN YOUR EYES TO THE WORLD AROUND YOU

Years ago, when I first practiced meditation, I would visualize myself walking through a gate and up some stairs to an outdoor room with the most amazing view of the expanse of the sea and the hills and trees surrounding it. As I entered that space, I felt so at ease and my life felt full of contentment.

Today, as the sun was setting in my home and I was finishing the final chapters of this book, I looked out of my window. I then had an epiphany. The vision of my perfect meditation place was right before me all the time, I just had not truly opened my eyes to see it because of always looking elsewhere for my peace or happiness. The outdoor room that I had visualized for all these years was my balcony overlooking the sea and the beautiful hills beyond.

In this moment I could not believe my eyes that, for years, the peace that I had been longing for was right in front of my eyes every single day. Through the busyness of my life, I had not opened my eyes properly to it and always thought that my peace was somewhere else. I just had not seen it in discontentment and in my search for more.

This is a problem for many. You can be so busy with life, constantly looking forward to the future, that you don't see that everything you need is right here, right now. The peace you are searching for is right in front of you, in this moment. You buy a house, then a few years later you want something bigger. You buy a nice dress then need another one because it has gone out of trend. We are constantly seeking that peace and happiness in new things, and that happiness is often short-lived when we actually receive what we want, as we then move on to an even bigger goal.

I talk about goals a lot in **The GLOW Ritual** and, as important as they are, it is also always important to know that your true happiness can always be found right here in this moment. Achieving your goals is the added bonus. We can often imprison ourselves in discontent for always wanting more and believing that our happiness lies in our future.

> *"The moment that judgement stops through acceptance of what is, your mind is free."*
> Eckhart Tolle - The Power of Now

Embrace your happiness today and open your eyes to your wonderful world around you.

THE YAMAS AND THE NIYAMAS

As mentioned previously, when I started to do my yoga teacher training in Philosophy and Ethical Practice, I discovered the ten guidelines of yoga – the Yamas and Niyamas – which can teach us a new way of living. Yoga is designed not just for the body, but for the mind too. The Yamas and Niyamas give us direction to live a joyous path.

The first five guidelines are referred to as Yamas, which

in Sanskrit translates to the word 'restraint'. These focus on how our adult relationship is with the world around us – our social focus.

These include:

Ahimsa – Non-violence
Satya – Truthfulness
Asteya – Non-stealing
Brahmacharya – Non-excess
Aparigraha – Non-possessiveness

The last five guidelines are referred to as the Niyamas, which in Sanskrit translates to 'observances' and is the adult relationship with ourselves – our inner focus.

These include:

Saucha – Purity
Santosha – Contentment
Tapas – Self-Discipline
Svadhyaya – Self-Study
Ishvara Pranidhana – Surrender

As I looked out of my window again, I remembered my teachings on *Santosha* – contentment. Within our materialistic society, we often find ourselves in discontent and always wanting more. Your neighbour might have a bigger house, a new designer bag has just been launched, your friend has won the lottery, your brother has just got a promotion… the list is endless. These things can lead us to become discontent with what we have because we always want more. We never live in the moment or arrive at our destination in pursuit of more because…

THERE IS ALWAYS MORE TO DESIRE.

BE CONTENT WITH WHERE YOU ARE

When we become content and grateful for what we have, we are never lacking and everything we get in the future is a bonus.

In one of my favourite books, *The Yamas & Niyamas* by Deborah Adele, she summarises the meaning of *Santosha* perfectly:

> *Santosha, or contentment, is performing duty and right action with pure joy. It is the true understanding that there is nothing more that can or does exist than this very moment.*

> *Discontentment is the illusion that there can be something else in the moment. There isn't and there can't be. The moment is complete.*

Being discontent with your life can block you from seeing that all you have desired is right in front of you.

Yoga teaches us the power of contentment as we are in the moments of flow on our mat. Our minds are not looking into the future, wishing for the perfect yoga body; they are in the moment, building our strength in the pose and our 100% focus on improving it. Yoga helps us to appreciate where we are now and how far we have come, not how far we have to go. It teaches us to not live in the future, but to be fully present without outside noise and grateful for where we are right now.

Sometimes you never appreciate what you have until it is gone. There will always be someone out there with more than you, and likewise there will be people out there less fortunate than you. However, we ALL have one unique life and so it is in OUR power to make the best of the life we have created for ourselves.

SWITCH FROM COMPARISON TO CONTENTMENT

Switch off from comparison and practice contentment. Switch off from scrolling through people's perceived 'perfect lives' and start living your own. When you are 90, you won't be wishing you had 10,000 followers on Instagram. You will be wishing that you had lived a life you loved and lived it to your fullest. So, why not begin your journey today of a life of gratitude and contentment and see the beauty that surrounds your life every day.

Contentment is being thankful and falling in love with your own life, not wishing you had someone else's.

FINDING PEACE IN THE PRESENT

Finding peace in the present can be so liberating because you let go of worry and remain relaxed about things that you cannot change. Meditation very much helps with this as it allows you to simply focus on the moment and not worry about the past or future.

As we approach the end of this book, I would like to allow you time to reflect on all you have learnt and how you can apply it to your life.

We find peace within ourselves when we are not on the hamster wheel of trying to impress people that do not matter or feeling like we are lacking in any way. We find our inner peace when we know that we have everything we need at hand and embrace a sense of calm in this present moment.

Over the years, I have practiced finding peace in the present more and more. I have gotten off the hamster wheel of pursuing and instead have been taking time to reflect how far I have come. You only appreciate where you are when you see how far you have come. When you are always looking into the future, you are no longer present. It is a gift in itself to be present in body, mind and spirit.

I still have goals in my life, many books that I want to get published and things that I want to do to learn and grow. However, I am peaceful knowing that things take time and that if I remain focused, I will achieve my goals. There is an inner peace when you have acceptance of your life path and how it will unfold.

So, as I leave you on the final chapter of this book, take time to reflect and make notes on what you will take away. What will be the changes that you make to live life a little more Zen and still achieve your goals? What mindset shifts can you make to help things happen without burning yourself out? There is peace that you will find within you when you find the pause button and know when you need to rest and reset. Never see taking time to pause as being at a standstill.

There are so many things you can achieve in your life with the knowledge that I have given you in *The GLOW Ritual*. My wish is that you achieve everything you want in your life by believing 100% that you can. Whether that is pursuing your dream career, creating more self-care rituals in your day, or just living a more peaceful and glowing life.

"In the end, only three things matter: how much you loved, how gently you lived, and how gracefully you let go of things not meant for you. All we are is the result of what we have thought."

Buddha

YOU CREATE YOUR OWN REALITY

What life will you start to create for yourself today?

This now leads us to **The GLOW Ritual for Contentment**...

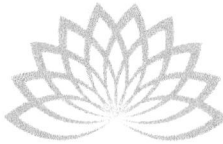

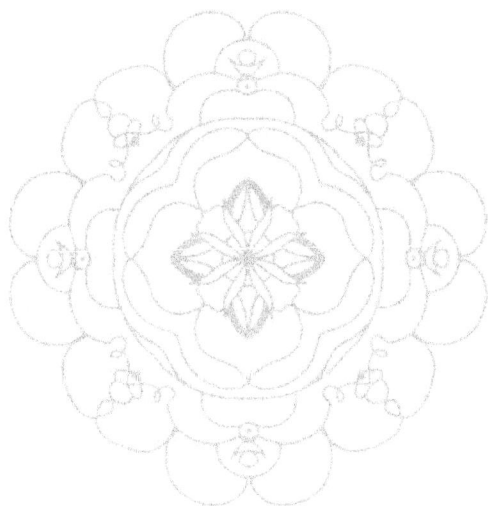

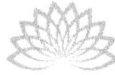

THE GLOW RITUAL
FOR CONTENTMENT

GRATITUDE & GET CREATIVE
Journaling Prompts

Today, write in your journal:

- How will you incorporate the Yamas and Niyamas into your daily life?
- Which one most resonated with you?
- What improvements would you like to see in your life?
- Write down 5 things that you are grateful for today

LIVE HOLISTICALLY
Life Lessons

- Be content with where you are right now
- Switch from comparison to contentment
- Find peace in the present moment
- You create your own reality
- Embrace your happiness today and open your eyes to your wonderful world around you

ORGANISE YOUR LIFE
Get Organised

Organise your thoughts of comparison to contentment. Organise your surroundings to reflect the life you want to live right now. Be present and at peace of where you are right now.

WELLNESS RITUALS
Time For Self-Care

Today, incorporate some of the Yamas and Niyamas into your way of living and see how much better you feel. Stop comparing yourself with others and be content in where you are. You create your own reality by pursuing your goals, not watching others achieve theirs. Focus on your journey.

I would love to see *The GLOW Ritual* you have decided to create for yourself today.

Don't forget to also tick each part of *The GLOW Ritual* off each day to support you in living your *Glowing Life Of Wellness*:

Gratitude & **G**et Creative
Live Holistically
Organise Your Life
Wellness Rituals

Share with me www.jaikooven.co.uk

DAY 31
THE GLOW RITUAL

*'Let The GLOW Ritual be your guiding
light back to wellness.'*
Jai Koo-Ven

DISCOVERING YOUR GLOW

I came up with the concept of *The GLOW Ritual* many years ago. Like a lot of people, I lacked confidence in 'putting my work out there', believing in myself that I could do it, and I also struggled to know how I could reach my goals. My aim from the beginning was that you, my reader, would have one place to go to provide you with the inspiration, motivation and positive guidance that you need when things get hard or overwhelming.

For a newbie on their journey to spirituality and wellness, you can feel very alone. You can feel scared of judgement from others and feel overwhelmed with where to start or how to get the support you need. I often felt overwhelmed when I first started too. Trying to understand my meditations from my mantras and confusion with my Chakras. My biggest struggle, however, was how to implement wellbeing rituals into my days in my busy world. This is why I created *The GLOW Ritual* and my membership programme. My mission has always been to make self-care simple for the busy modern woman and to encourage women to create a life they love.

I hope that *The GLOW Ritual* has provided you with an easy introduction into the wellness world and how it can benefit your life a little each day. As I mentioned before, during the creation of this book I also developed The Mind Spa Membership – an online wellness membership for the busy modern woman and your Self-Care Sanctuary for your daily wellbeing. You can gain access to this when you work 1:1 with me through my wellbeing programme. The membership is great to use in addition to this book. I hope that my book, membership and 1:1 consultations give you plenty of support that you need to up-level your wellbeing and live your best life.

I have learnt how important wellbeing rituals are in my life over the years and the need to keep them at the top of my to-do list every day. When you look after your wellbeing, you can up-level your life in so many different ways. You are able to create success for yourself because you can take time out and assess when things are not working for you and find another way.

We all have the same 24-hours as everyone else, so why is it that some people achieve so much more than others in their day and in their lives? There are two simple answers for this: the successful people plan and implement what they learn, and they apply it to their days. It is my hope that you take the lessons that I have taught you and apply them to your life each day. We all get overwhelmed at times with busy schedules and endless to-do lists. Even as I write the end of this book, we have gone into our third national lockdown in the UK, and my daughter is currently being home-schooled because the schools are shut. However, when crisis and chaos hits, we just need to adapt to the situation and do the next thing that will make a difference and guide ourselves back to calm. Be proactive rather than reactive. This is the only way that you will move forward to creating the life of your dreams.

FIND YOUR INNER GLOW

I am so thankful for you making my dream come true. All

I ever wanted with writing this book was to make people feel supported, comforted, and feel like they are not alone on their wellbeing journey. I hope that I was able to create a special support for you and keep you focused on the light. There is light in every dark scenario and always a lesson to learn.

Let **The GLOW Ritual** always be your guiding light back to a **Glowing Life of Wellness**:

G – GRATITUDE & GET CREATIVE

Be grateful for all that you have and all that you are. Express your creativity each day to boost your happiness and focus. Use your creative energy to inspire you to create a beautiful life.

L – LIVE HOLISTICALLY

Apply the holistic guidance from **The GLOW Ritual** to create a healthy balance of your body, mind and spirit. Living holistically is a luxury that is worth your investment each day.

O – ORGANISE YOUR LIFE

Feeling overwhelmed? Then the first thing to do is to get organised. Messy house, messy mind. So, declutter your space and it will declutter your mind to help you think more clearly.

W – WELLNESS RITUALS

Welcome wellness rituals in your daily life, no matter whether you have 5-minutes or two hours. Create a wonderful sacred space where you feel calm and spend time meditating and journaling to release negative energy, boost your positivity, and reflect on what you want from of your life. Use the 31 Wellness Rituals in this book to guide you whenever you need extra support.

We all have the power to change our scenarios, thoughts and feelings every day. Many of us dwell too much on what we can't change, rather than focus on what we can change. Or we get so overwhelmed that we just do not start. Take back your power and know that you have a choice each day to live a life you love. It is never too late to start again. Always keep trying and never give up.

GLOW IN EVERY MOMENT

See the good in each and every scenario and learn that there is always a way forward, even though at the time you may feel stuck.

Everything we go through in life is to help us glow, grow and get stronger. We adapt, we change and we springboard ourselves to the next level.

I hope, whether you are embracing a more holistic life or going through the hustle of building your new business, that I have inspired you to put yourself out there and not be afraid to show the world your greatness.

Daily self-care goes beyond just having a bit of 'me time'. Self-care feeds our soul, allows us to make time for ourselves to relax, reflect and feel good. Take time for that each day and remember that your self-care should always be at your top of your list. When your cup is empty, what do you have to give to yourself or anyone else?

'When you know your worth, you do not have to prove to anyone the luxury of you.

Let THE GLOW RITUAL spark a fire within you to ignite your greatness, make the impossible possible and guide you to living an abundant and GLOWING LIFE OF WELLNESS.'

With Love & Light,

Jai Koo-Ven

So, this now leads us to your final **GLOW Ritual**…

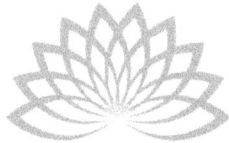

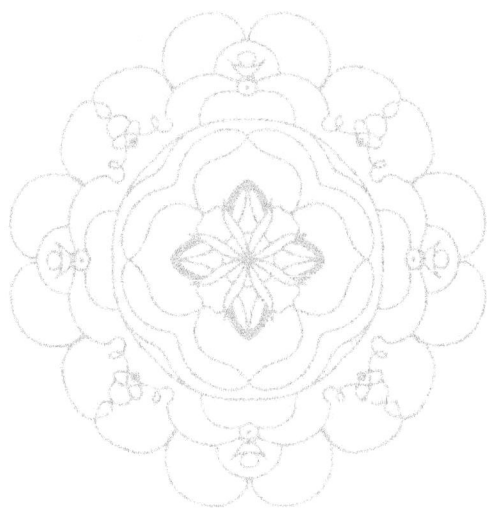

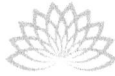

THE GLOW RITUAL

GRATITUDE & GET CREATIVE
Journaling Prompts

Today, write in your journal:

- List 10 things you are grateful for
- What has bought you the most joy today?
- What about yourself are you grateful for?
- Write down 5 things you are grateful for today

LIVE HOLISTICALLY
Life Lessons

- Let *The GLOW Ritual* ignite the fire within you to go after the life that you want
- See the good in every scenario and learn that there is always a way forward, even though at the time you may feel stuck
- Apply the holistic guidance from *The GLOW Ritual* to create a healthy balance of your body, mind and spirit
- Living holistically is a luxury that is worth your investment each day

ORGANISE YOUR LIFE
Get Organised

With all the Wellness Rituals that you have tried in this book, now get organised and create your own wellness ritual which you can stick to on a daily basis that will help you maintain a clutter-free home and a healthy and happy body and mind.

WELLNESS RITUALS
Time For Self-Care

Today, whatever is going on in your life, be grateful for everything you have and everything you have received. Show your gratitude to someone by writing them a letter, taking them out for the day or treating them to something nice. When you practice having gratitude, you can receive more in abundance. When you are not grateful, less comes to you. Find moments every day to incorporate *The GLOW Ritual* into your life.

I would love to see *The GLOW Ritual* you have decided to create for yourself today.

Don't forget to also tick each part of *The GLOW Ritual* off each day to support you in living your *Glowing Life Of Wellness*:

Gratitude & **G**et Creative
Live Holistically
Organise Your Life
Wellness Rituals

Share with me www.jaikooven.co.uk

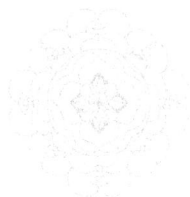

THE CROWN CHAKRA RITUAL

In this chapter, we covered:

- *The GLOW Ritual* for Calm
- *The GLOW Ritual* for Contentment
- *The GLOW Ritual*

This chapter provided the building blocks to help you discover how you can create calm in a chaotic life and make time for peace and gratitude. We covered how meditation can help you find moments of stillness and calm in your day. You also learnt how you have the power to create your own reality and live a life of peace and contentment through the yoga philosophy of the *Yamas* and *Niyamas*.

REFLECTION

When you look at your current life now, what could you change for a more positive life? We reflected on *The GLOW Ritual* self-discovery journey. What rituals will you continue from the teachings that you have learnt from this book?

POSITIVE CHANGE

You can create any life you want with the correct mindset and focus. Your positive change going forwards is to consistently try to improve yourself every day, no matter how big or small.

CRYSTALS FOR CROWN CHAKRA

Amethyst

Amethyst helps relieve stress and soothe irritability. It helps to balance mood swings and anger and also helps with anxiety and grief. It is great at dissolving negativity. Amethyst is a fabulous spiritual support crystal that will aid you in tapping into your intuition.

Clear Quartz

Clear Quartz is great at focusing the mind and bringing clarity into your life.

White Agate

White Agate is a beautiful crystal for balance and release. It supports you with any mental issues, including frustration and anxiety. It is fantastic for stimulating the Crown Chakra and is often used for worry stones.

ESSENTIAL OILS FOR THE CROWN CHAKRA

Use an essential oil diffuser to surround yourself with a choice of one of these scents or create your own uplifting mixture.

PLEASE SEEK MEDICAL OR PROFESSIONAL ADVICE IF YOU ARE PREGNANT OR HAVE A MEDICAL CONDITION.

Rosemary

If you want to take action, then rosemary is said to improve your memory. It is great if you are starting a new venture or learning something new.

Lavender

Lavender is a great multi-purpose essential oil which is known for its calming and relaxing properties. If you need time to rest and retreat, this essential oil will provide you with lovely moments of calm.

Fennel

Fennel is great for supporting you both spiritually and emotionally. It can help with motivation, self-confidence and can support you in living and authentic life in line with your values.

Well done on completing your last Chakra Chapter.

I would love to see *The GLOW Ritual* you have decided to create for yourself today.

Don't forget to also tick each part of *The GLOW Ritual* off each day to support you in living your *Glowing Life Of Wellness*:

Gratitude & **G**et Creative
Live Holistically
Organise Your Life
Wellness Rituals

Share with me www.jaikooven.co.uk

GLOW WITH GRATITUDE

I am so thankful for this most amazing opportunity. It is everything I could have wished for and I am grateful for the support that I have received in turning my words into *The GLOW Ritual*.

Thank you to Sean at That Guy's House for helping me turn my dream into a physical product and listening to my crazy ideas. I am so blessed to be working with you to create this book.

Thank you to Martina, my talented illustrator. You took my ideas and created my vision through your art. I am so grateful to you for creating such a beautiful design and I have loved working with you on my projects. Thank you for being amazing and very patient.

Thanks to Emma Mumford for mentoring me through the 'birthing' process of this book. I am so grateful for your knowledge and expertise to keep me on track and inspiring me to keep on going.

Thank you to the holistic world for giving me the knowledge that I needed to heal myself, learn and grow. It is my hope that it will help and inspire people all over the world.

Thank you to my dear late stepdad, Graham, for always believing in me. This book is dedicated to you, and I hope wherever you are at this moment, you are looking down at me, smiling and very proud. I promised you I would do it, and my promise to you kept me going when times were hard. You are and always will be my guardian angel who will always make me believe that the impossible is always possible. Thank you for always believing in me and showing me that I can. I love you so much and am so thankful for our time together on this earth.

Thank you to my amazing husband and daughter for putting up with my constant ideas, moments of silence and late-night writing processes. I appreciate your support during a time that really mattered to me. I could not have done this without your love and constant support and patience during this time.

I love you both very much. xx

Lastly, thank you to you, my reader. This is all for you. Thank you so much for choosing my book out of all the millions of books out there. I am so grateful that it inspired you to take a read. Use *The GLOW Ritual* whenever you need some guidance or a pick me up and visit my website www.jaikooven.co.uk if you would like any further support. You can also follow me on Instagram @jaikooven_.

I would love to support you and help you create your own beautiful *Glowing Life Of Wellness*.

Love,

Jai x

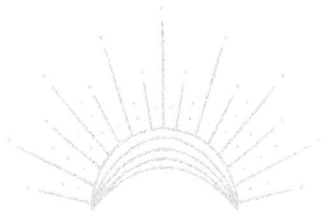

Crystal & Essential Oil

MINI GUIDE

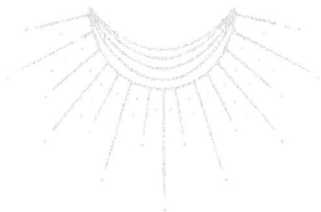

MINI CRYSTAL & ESSENTIAL OIL GUIDE

You may have heard about healing crystals but did not know the benefits that they could have on you. There are a huge number of crystals with various healing abilities that you can use to help you with your daily emotions as well as physical and spiritual benefits. They can also help a lot with emotions such as anxiety and depression. Crystal healing has been used for centuries to help treat the mind, body *and* spirit holistically.

When buying a crystal, go for one that you feel most drawn to as this is a guide that you need this particular energy at this time. I have a variety in my online boutique www.jaikooven.co.uk

On the following pages I have created a Crystal & Essential Oils Guide for your Chakras and also a Mini Crystal Guide for your wellbeing to reference whenever you need to.

CRYSTALS & ESSENTIAL OILS FOR THE ROOT CHAKRA:

Red Jasper
Red jasper is the overall crystal balancer for this Chakra as it is the supreme nurturer and stone of endurance.

Moss Agate
Moss agate is known as the 'stabilizer stone'. It helps with supportive growth. It has loving Earth energy to assist you steadily enduring anything that life throws at you. It gives you confidence of Mother Earth as you concentrate and focus on attracting financial prosperity and business success.

Blue Lace Agate
One of my favourite crystals is blue lace agate which is a variety of chalcedony. Not only does it look beautiful, but it will also give you a wonderful feeling of calm and help guide you back to happiness.

Citrine
Keep citrine in your wallet or purse and in your office as this attracts wealth and abundance.

ESSENTIAL OILS FOR THE ROOT CHAKRA

Use an essential oil diffuser to surround yourself with a choice of one of these scents or create your own uplifting mixture.

PLEASE SEEK MEDICAL OR PROFESSIONAL ADVICE IF YOU ARE PREGNANT OR HAVE A MEDICAL CONDITION.

Lemon is uplifting and enhances a positive mood.

Ginger root is energizing and grounding.

Peppermint prevents fatigue and improves exercise performance.

Pine provides a boost of energy levels.

Ylang ylang reduces depression and boosts your mood.

CRYSTALS & ESSENTIAL OILS FOR THE SACRAL CHAKRA

Carnelian
Carnelian is the overall crystal balancer for this Chakra as it is a great crystal for motivation and creativity. It encourages us to embrace vitality in our lives by living in the present moment.

Sunstone
Sunstone is great for boosting your self-confidence and boosting your Sacral and Solar Plexus Chakras and supporting you with strength and enthusiasm in your new goals.

Citrine
Citrine helps to give you joyful energy and makes you feel more positive. It is also a great crystal for attracting abundance.

ESSENTIAL OILS FOR THE SACRAL CHAKRA:

Use an essential oil diffuser to surround yourself with a choice of one of these scents or create your own uplifting mixture.

PLEASE SEEK MEDICAL OR PROFESSIONAL ADVICE IF YOU ARE PREGNANT OR HAVE A MEDICAL CONDITION.

Sweet Orange Oil

Sweet orange oil is great for making you feel uplifted and happy. It is refreshing and encourages fun, joy and creativity as it is also known as the 'Smiley Oil'.

Jasmine

Jasmine is a great essential oil for confidence and optimism. It brings a sense of euphoria to your mind and helps you feel more confident when tackling larger projects.

Frankincense

Frankincense is the essential oil for calming and soothing the mind, body and spirit. It is a nurturing oil that allows us to gain creative clarity.

CRYSTALS & ESSENTIAL OILS FOR THE SOLAR PLEXUS CHAKRA

Amazonite

Amazonite is one of my favourite crystals Not only is it beautiful to look at, but it allows us to enjoy happier relationships and tune into our intuition. It also allows us to make healthier decisions that can lead to our overall happiness.

Citrine

Citrine helps to give you joyful energy and makes you feel more positive. It is also a great crystal for attracting abundance.

Amethyst

Amethyst is a beautiful and calming crystal. It helps to keep us centred whilst also uplifting us.

ESSENTIAL OILS FOR THE SOLAR PLEXUS CHAKRA

Use an essential oil diffuser to surround yourself with a choice of one of these scents or create your own uplifting mixture.

PLEASE SEEK MEDICAL OR PROFESSIONAL ADVICE IF YOU ARE PREGNANT OR HAVE A MEDICAL CONDITION.

Lavender
Lavender essential oil is very popular for relaxation; however, it also has an uplifting effect that boosts your overall happiness levels. It also helps with anxiety and stress.

Bergamot
Bergamot essential oil is great for supporting you in alleviating work-related stress by reducing feelings of anxiety and making you feel more relaxed and happier.

Jasmine
Jasmine is one of my favourite essential oils and is really popular in perfumes. Jasmine promotes a wonderful feeling of wellbeing and happiness. It also makes you feel more romantic and energetic.

CRYSTALS & ESSENTIAL OILS FOR THE PINK HEART CHAKRA

Pink Tourmaline
Pink tourmaline will help to calm down the skin and soothe it by maintaining moisture within the skin. It also promotes harmony and calms the mind.

Rose Quartz
Rose quartz is a gorgeous crystal with multiple benefits, one of them being that it soothes the heart with it gentle, loving and heart-focused loving energy. This crystal is great for heartbreak through a divorce, breakup or bereavement.

Amethyst
Amethyst is great to support you during the grieving process as it can help promote dreaming and work with your subconscious, so you may dream about your loved one.

ESSENTIAL OILS FOR THE PINK HEART CHAKRA

Use an essential oil diffuser to surround yourself with a choice of one of these scents or create your own uplifting mixture.

PLEASE SEEK MEDICAL OR PROFESSIONAL ADVICE IF YOU ARE PREGNANT OR HAVE A MEDICAL CONDITION.

Rose
This is a great essential oil for self-love. It is a very comforting and nurturing scent that supports the Heart Chakra.

Patchouli
Patchouli is great at supporting you with feelings of depression and bereavement.

Chamomile
Chamomile is a beautiful essential oil which is not only calming but uplifting too. It can also support you in having a restful sleep.

CRYSTALS & ESSENTIAL OILS FOR THE GREEN HEART CHAKRA

Tiger's Eye
Tiger's eye is great for focus and determination – great if you want to take action.

Clear Quartz
Clear quartz is wonderful for focusing the mind and bringing clarity into your life or knowing whether you need to take action or rest.

Blue Lace Agate
Blue lace agate helps you to feel calm and relaxed when you need some time out.

ESSENTIAL OILS FOR THE GREEN HEART CHAKRA

Use an essential oil diffuser to surround yourself with a choice of one of these scents or create your own uplifting mixture.

PLEASE SEEK MEDICAL OR PROFESSIONAL ADVICE IF YOU ARE PREGNANT OR HAVE A MEDICAL CONDITION.

Rosemary
If you want to take action, then rosemary is said to improve your memory, so it is great if you are starting a new venture or learning something new.

Lavender
Lavender is a great multi-purpose essential oil which is known for its calming and relaxing properties. If you need time to rest and retreat, this essential oil will provide you with lovely moments of calm.

Grapefruit

If you are coming out of your Yin phase and feel the need to be more energised, then grapefruit would be perfect for you as it has a beautiful and uplifting fragrance which helps to give your mind and body an energy boost.

CRYSTALS & ESSENTIAL OILS FOR THE THROAT CHAKRA

Tiger's Eye

Tiger's Eye is great for focus and determination and is helpful for writers on a self-healing journey.

Clear Quartz

Clear quartz helps with focusing the mind and bringing clarity into your life.

Blue Lace Agate

Blue lace agate is beneficial for stimulating communication in your life and supporting you in feeling calm and relaxed. This crystal is wonderful in supporting you to speak your truth.

ESSENTIAL OILS FOR THE THROAT CHAKRA

Use an essential oil diffuser to surround yourself with a choice of one of these scents or create your own uplifting mixture.

PLEASE SEEK MEDICAL OR PROFESSIONAL ADVICE IF YOU ARE PREGNANT OR HAVE A MEDICAL CONDITION.

Rosemary

Rosemary essential oil is known to improve brain function and memory. So, this a great essential oil to use whilst you are cross-referencing information as it allows you to stay focused during the process.

Lavender
Lavender is a fabulous multi-purpose essential oil which is known for its calming and relaxing properties. If you are writing in your journal about something difficult or have to do public speaking, it can be quite stressful – this essential oil will help to keep you calm during this time.

Wild Orange
Wild orange essential oil is really uplifting and can provide a huge amount of emotional and spiritual support which can help you manifest your desires.

CRYSTALS & ESSENTIAL OILS FOR THE THIRD EYE CHAKRA

Use an essential oil diffuser to surround yourself with a choice of one of these scents or create your own uplifting mixture:

CRYSTALS FOR THIRD EYE CHAKRA

Lapis Lazuli
This crystal looks so beautiful with its gorgeous blue hue. It helps to block negative energy and allows positivity to flow to you.

Clear Quartz
Clear quartz is great at focusing the mind and bringing clarity into your life.

Snowflake Obsidian
This crystal is calming and soothing, providing peace and balance in the mind, body and spirit. It recognizes

your uniqueness and your individuality. It will remove feelings of isolation if you are alone, allowing you to remain confident and secure and encouraging you to be your true self

ESSENTIAL OILS FOR THE THIRD EYE CHAKRA

Use an essential oil diffuser to surround yourself with a choice of one of these scents or create your own uplifting mixture.

PLEASE SEEK MEDICAL OR PROFESSIONAL ADVICE IF

YOU ARE PREGNANT OR HAVE A MEDICAL CONDITION.

Frankincense
Frankincense is the perfect essential oil for calming and soothing the mind, body and spirit. It is a nurturing oil that allows us to gain creative clarity.

Basil
Basil is great for stimulating, calming, energising, clarifying and uplifting the mind. It can also soothe headaches and eliminate odour-causing bacteria as well as repel insects.

Fennel
Fennel is wonderful for supporting you both spiritually and emotionally. It can help with motivation, self-confidence and can support you in living an authentic life in line with your values.

CRYSTALS & ESSENTIAL OILS FOR THE CROWN CHAKRA

Amethyst

Amethyst helps relieve stress and soothe irritability. It helps to balance mood swings and anger and also helps with anxiety and grief. It is great at dissolving negativity. Amethyst is a fabulous spiritual support crystal that will aid you in tapping into your intuition.

Clear Quartz

Clear quartz is great at focusing the mind and bringing clarity into your life.

White Agate

White agate is a beautiful crystal for balance and release. It supports you with any mental issues, including frustration and anxiety. It is fantastic for stimulating the Crown Chakra and is often used for worry stones.

ESSENTIAL OILS FOR THE CROWN CHAKRA

Use an essential oil diffuser to surround yourself with a choice of one of these scents or create your own uplifting mixture.

PLEASE SEEK MEDICAL OR PROFESSIONAL ADVICE IF YOU ARE PREGNANT OR HAVE A MEDICAL CONDITION.

Rosemary

If you want to take action, then rosemary is said to improve your memory, so it is great if you are starting a new venture or learning something new.

Lavender
Lavender is a great multi-purpose essential oil which is known for its calming and relaxing properties. If you need time to rest and retreat, this essential oil will provide you with lovely moments of calm.

Fennel
Fennel is great for supporting you both spiritually and emotionally. It can help with motivation, self-confidence and can support you in living and authentic life in line with your values.

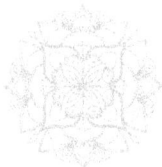

CRYSTALS FOR YOUR WELLBEING

Here are some crystals that I recommend for your wellbeing:

CRYSTALS FOR HAPPINESS

Amazonite
Amazonite is one of my favourite crystals and is beautiful to look at. This crystal helps us to feel empowered, enjoy happier relationships and let go of your limiting beliefs.

Amethyst
Amethyst is great for grief but also for happiness as it helps to keep you calm and centred, and it also keeps you uplifted.

Ametrine

A combination of amethyst and citrine, ametrine gives you the best of both worlds, as it provides you with joy and calm. It also promotes optimism and clarity and supports positive change in your life.

CRYSTALS FOR A DIGITAL DETOX

Himalayan Salt Lamps – These are beautiful as home décor as well as believed to have various health benefits. They can help with asthma as well as detoxing a room. They release helpful negative ions into the room and clean the air.

Shungite – This is an ancient crystal which is said to protect you from EMF, as it contains fullerenes. These allow this crystal to magnetise, neutralise and destroy free radicals while remaining intact. It is a very powerful absorbing stone. Also, a great grounding stone for the Root Chakra.

Pyrite - Do not place this crystal too close to any devices as it can cause issues with their performance. Pyrite works by absorbing and dampening the EMF frequencies.

CRYSTALS FOR GROUNDING & PROTECTION

Moss Agate – This is a lovely crystal that symbolises new beginnings. It is a great crystal for self-expression and communication. Moss agate helps you to balance your emotions, which help release fear and stress. It encourages hope and trust in your life and eliminates depression caused by imbalances in your brain.

Amber – Amber is regarded as a stone of courage and was considered the 'soul of the tiger' in Asian cultures. Amber was often carried for protection during long travels. It is a great crystal to attract good luck and balance emotions.

CRYSTALS FOR CREATING CALM

Kyanite – This is a beautifully coloured crystal which helps with meditation and attunement. Kyanite helps to align all your Chakras. It provides you with the perfect balance of yin-yang energy, moves energy gently through your body and helps to eliminate blockages. Kyanite brings tranquillity and calm to your whole being.

Rose Quartz – Beautiful loving energy. This is the stone of universal love. It restores harmony and trust in relationships. It purifies and opens up your heart at all levels to promote self-love, deep inner healing and feelings of peace.

CRYSTALS FOR MANIFESTATION

Malachite – Malachite is a lovely stone of abundance, balance, setting intentions and manifestations. It is a really powerful metaphysical stone and is often called the 'Stone of Transformation'. It gives out deep energy cleaning which can bring healing and positive transformation to you.

Magnetite – Magnetite is a great crystal for manifestation and can help you attract what you most desire in life or with people. It is also known as the Lodestone. Magnetite is naturally magnetic.

CRYSTALS FOR ATTRACTING MONEY

Citrine – Keep citrine in your wallet or purse and in your office as this attracts wealth and abundance.

Peridot can help you see into the future and help you make smarter financial decisions. It also acts as a wealth magnet.

Black Tourmaline is one of the best crystals for debt. It helps to awaken your mind by clearing the clutter rationally.

Pyrite helps with prosperity and is one of the best abundance stones that will help you to regain financial balance. It keeps attracting prosperity and protects you from debt.

CRYSTALS FOR A HAPPY HOME

Rose Quartz – Place in your bedroom to surround yourself with love.

Black Onyx – Place near your front door to keep out negative energies.

Golden Citrine – Place in your office to attract abundance and success.

Clear Quartz – Place in the bathroom to cleanse the soul daily.

Purple Amethyst – Place in a busy room to promote tranquillity and calm.

CRYSTALS TO FOR SACRED SPACES

Rose Quartz – Beautiful loving energy. This is the stone of universal love. It restores harmony and trust in relationships. It purifies and opens up your heart at all levels to promote self-love, deep inner healing and feelings of peace.

Turquoise – This is one of my favourite crystals as it is a purification stone which balances and aligns all the Chakras and helps stabilise moods swings. It also gives you a strong sense of inner calm when you are in its presence. It is great for exhaustion or depression and has the power to prevent panic attacks. Turquoise is also a great stone for assisting with creative problem-solving and self-realisation.

Selenite – A powerful cleansing stone. Helps you connect to your higher self by balancing your Third Eye and Crown Chakras. It draws white light down from the astral plan and into our physical world.

Black Tourmaline – Great for placing at the entrance of the sacred space. It acts as a protective guardian, keeping out bad vibes. It will keep good energy flowing around the space and establish a sense of balance.

CRYSTALS FOR INNER CHILD HEALING

Amazonite
Amazonite is one of my favourite crystals and is beautiful to look at. This crystal helps us to feel empowered, enjoy happier relationships and let go of your limiting beliefs.

Amethyst
Amethyst is great for grief but also for happiness as it helps to keep you calm and centred, and it also keeps you uplifted.

Ametrine

You experience the best of both worlds with Ametrine as it provides you with joy and calm. It also promotes optimism and clarity and supports positive change in your life.

REFERENCES

Wikipedia.org

Headspace

Brainyquote.com

Healthline.com

Quotestates.com

Proflowers.com

Californiapsychics.com

Cosmiccuts.com

Kaliana.com

Yogajournal.com

Craftsy.com

Betterhelp.com

Dying.lovetoknow.com

Stillpointaromatics.com

Spiritualityhealth.com

Theminimalists.com

Monq.com

Mindbodygreen.com

The Crystal Bible by Judy Hall

Crystals by Katie by Jane Wright

What I Know for Sure by Oprah Winfrey

The Ayurvedic Self-Care Handbook by Sarah Kucera

The Secret by Rhonda Byrne

The Yamas & Niyamas by Deborah Adele

The War of Art – Steven Pressfield

The Universe Has Your Back – Gabrielle Bernstein

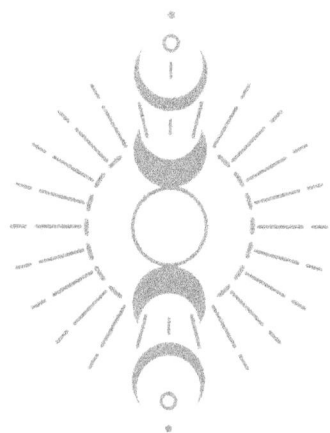

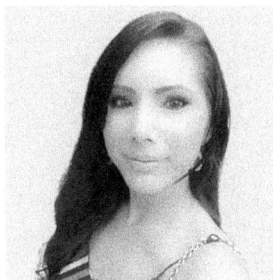

ABOUT THE AUTHOR

JAI KOO-VEN is an Author, International Holistic Expert and owner of her own wellbeing clinic for women. She is also the designer behind her own Self-Care Stationery and wellness brand.

Jai is passionate about encouraging you to be inspired each day to become the best version of you and make time for your wellbeing.

When she is not writing books, reading and working with clients, you will find her in the aisles of her favourite bookshops finding inspiration for her next book.

Visit www.jaikooven.co.uk or follow her on Instagram @jaikooven_

Lightning Source UK Ltd.
Milton Keynes UK
UKHW022251120822
407231UK00003B/17